# MEDICAL
# STATISTICS
# MADE EASY **3**

# OTHER TITLES FROM SCION

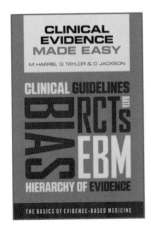
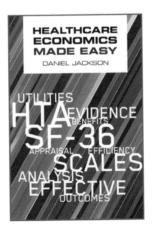
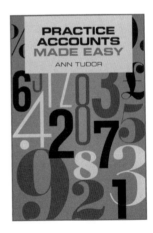

For more information see www.scionpublishing.com

# MEDICAL STATISTICS MADE EASY 3

**Michael Harris**

*Associate Postgraduate Dean Emeritus and former General Practitioner, Bristol, UK*

*and*

**Gordon Taylor**

*Reader in Medical Statistics, University of Bath, UK*

Scion

KH

**Third edition © Scion Publishing Ltd, 2014**

ISBN 978 1 907904 03 5

Second edition published in 2008 by Scion Publishing Ltd (978 1 904842 55 2)

First edition published in 2003 by Martin Dunitz (1 85996 219 X)

**Scion Publishing Limited**

The Old Hayloft, Vantage Business Park, Bloxham Road, Banbury OX16 9UX, UK

www.scionpublishing.com

Typeset by Phoenix Photosetting, Chatham, Kent, UK

Printed by Charlesworth Press, Wakefield, UK

6/3/15

# CONTENTS

# ABBREVIATIONS

| | |
|---|---|
| ARR | absolute risk reduction |
| BMI | body mass index |
| BP | blood pressure |
| CI | confidence interval |
| df | degrees of freedom |
| HR | hazard ratio |
| ICC | intra-class correlation coefficient |
| IQR | inter-quartile range |
| LR | likelihood ratio |
| NNH | number needed to harm |
| NNT | number needed to treat |
| NPV | negative predictive value |
| $P$ | probability |
| PPV | positive predictive value |
| RRR | relative risk reduction |
| SD | standard deviation |

# PREFACE

This book is designed for healthcare students and professionals who need a basic knowledge of when common statistical terms are used and what they mean.

Whether you love or hate statistics, you need to have some understanding of the subject if you want to critically appraise a paper. To do this, you *do not* need to know how to do a statistical analysis. What you *do* need is to know why the test has been used and how to interpret the resulting figures.

This book does not assume that you have any prior statistical knowledge. However basic your mathematical or statistical knowledge, you will find that everything is clearly explained.

A few readers will find some of the sections ridiculously simplistic, others will find some bafflingly difficult. The "thumbs up" grading will help you pick out concepts that suit your level of understanding.

The "star" system is designed to help you pick out the most important concepts if you are short of time.

This book is also produced for those who may be asked about statistics in an exam. Pick out the "exam tips" sections if you are in a hurry.

You can test your understanding of what you have learnt by working through extracts from original papers in the "Statistics at work" section.

# ABOUT THE AUTHORS

Dr Michael Harris MB BS FRCGP MMEd is Associate Postgraduate Dean Emeritus, Bristol, UK. As well as being a General Practitioner, his roles have included medical education and being an examiner for the MRCGP.

Dr Gordon Taylor PhD MSc BSc (Hons) is a Reader in Medical Statistics at the University of Bath, UK. His main role is in the teaching, support and supervision of health care professionals involved in non-commercial research.

# FOREWORD

A love of statistics is, oddly, not what attracts most young people to a career in medicine and I suspect that many clinicians, like me, have at best a sketchy and incomplete understanding of this difficult subject.

Delivering modern, high quality care to patients now relies increasingly on routine reference to scientific papers and journals, rather than traditional textbook learning. Acquiring the skills to appraise medical research papers is a daunting task. Realizing this, Michael Harris and Gordon Taylor have expertly constructed a practical guide for the busy clinician. One an experienced NHS doctor, the other a medical statistician with a tremendous track record in clinical research, they have produced a unique handbook. It is short, readable and useful, without becoming overly bogged down in the mathematical detail that frankly puts so many of us off the subject.

I commend this book to all healthcare students and professionals, general practitioners and hospital specialists. It covers all the ground necessary to critically evaluate the statistical elements of medical research papers, in a friendly and approachable way. The scoring of each brief chapter in terms of usefulness and ease of comprehension will efficiently guide the busy practitioner through his or her reading.

In particular it is almost unique in covering this part of the syllabus for Royal College and other postgraduate examinations. Certainly a candidate familiar with the contents of this short book and taking note of its numerous helpful examination tips should have few difficulties when answering the questions on statistics in the Applied Knowledge Test module of the MRCGP exam.

March 2014
Prof Bill Irish
BSc MB BChir DCH DRCOG MMEd FRCGP
(GP Dean, Health Education South West, and Chairman, Committee of GP Education Directors, UK)

## Ch 1    HOW TO USE THIS BOOK

You can use this book in a number of ways.

### If you want a statistics course

- Work through from start to finish for a complete course in commonly used medical statistics.

### If you are in a hurry

- Choose the sections with the most stars to learn about the commonest statistical methods and terms.

- You may wish to start with these 5-star sections: percentages (*Chapter 3*), mean (*Chapter 4*), standard deviation (*Chapter 7*), confidence intervals (*Chapter 8*) and P values (*Chapter 9*).

### If you are daunted by statistics

- If you are bewildered every time someone tries to explain a statistical method, then pick out the sections with the most thumbs up symbols to find the easiest and most basic concepts.

- You may want to start with percentages (*Chapter 3*), mean (*Chapter 4*), median (*Chapter 5*) and mode (*Chapter 6*), then move on to risk ratio (*Chapter 13*), incidence and prevalence (in *Chapter 22*).

## If you are taking an exam

- The "Exam Tips" give you pointers to the topics which examiners like to ask about.

- You will find these in the following sections: mean (*Chapter 4*), standard deviation (*Chapter 7*), confidence intervals (*Chapter 8*), P values (*Chapter 9*), risk reduction and NNT (*Chapter 15*), sensitivity, specificity and predictive value (*Chapter 20*), incidence and prevalence (in *Chapter 22*).

## Test your understanding

- See how statistical methods are used in five extracts from real-life papers in the "Statistics at work" section (*Chapters 23–28*).

- Work out which statistical methods have been used, why, and what the results mean. Then check your understanding in our commentaries.

## Glossary

- Use the *Glossary* as a quick reference for statistical words or phrases that you do not know.

## Study advice

- Go through difficult sections when you are fresh and try not to cover too much at once.

- You may need to read some sections a couple of times before the meaning sinks in. You will find that the examples help you to understand the principles.

- We have tried to cut down the jargon as much as possible. If there is a word that you do not understand, check it out in the *Glossary*.

# Ch 2   HOW THIS BOOK IS DESIGNED

Every section uses the same series of headings to help you understand the concepts.

## "How important is it?"

We noted how often statistical terms were used in 200 quantitative papers in mainstream medical journals. All the papers selected for this survey were published during the last year in the *British Medical Journal*, *The Lancet*, *BJU International*, the *New England Journal of Medicine* and the *Journal of the American Medical Association*.

We grouped the terms into concepts and graded them by how often they were used. This helped us to develop a star system for importance. We also took into account usefulness to readers. For example, "numbers needed to treat" are not often quoted but are fairly easy to calculate and useful in making treatment decisions.

✪✪✪✪✪     Concepts which are used in the majority of medical papers.

✪✪✪✪     Important concepts which are used in at least a third of papers.

✪✪✪     Less frequently used, but still of value in decision-making.

✪✪          Found in at least 1 in 10 papers.

✪           Rarely used in medical journals.

## How easy is it to understand?

We have found that the ability of health care professionals to understand statistical concepts varies more widely than their ability to understand anything else related to medicine. This ranges from those that have no difficulty learning how to understand regression to those that struggle with percentages.

One of the authors (not the statistician!) fell into the latter category. He graded each section by how easy it is to understand the concept.

👍👍👍👍👍    Even the most statistic-phobic will have little difficulty in understanding these sections.

👍👍👍👍    With a little concentration, most readers should be able to follow these concepts.

👍👍👍    Some readers will have difficulty following these. You may need to go over these sections a few times to be able to take them in.

👍👍    Quite difficult to understand. Only tackle these sections when you are fresh.

👍    Statistical concepts that are very difficult to grasp.

## When is it used?

One thing you need to do if critically appraising a paper is check that the right statistical technique has been used. This part explains which statistical method should be used for what scenario.

## What does it mean?

This explains the bottom line – what the results mean and what to look out for to help you interpret them.

## Examples

Sometimes the best way to understand a statistical technique is to work through an example. Simple, fictitious examples are given to illustrate the principles and how to interpret them.

## Watch out for ...

This includes more detailed explanation, tips and common pitfalls.

## Exam tips

Some topics are particularly popular with examiners because they test understanding and involve simple calculations. We have given tips on how to approach these concepts.

# Ch 3    PERCENTAGES

## How important are they?

✪✪✪✪✪ An understanding of percentages is probably the first and most important concept to understand in statistics!

## How easy are they to understand?

👍👍👍👍👍 Percentages are easy to understand.

## When are they used?

Percentages are mainly used in the tabulation of data in order to give the reader a scale on which to assess or compare the data.

## What do they mean?

"Per cent" means per hundred, so a percentage describes a proportion of 100. For example 50% is 50 out of 100, or as a fraction ½. Other common percentages are 25% (25 out of 100 or ¼) and 75% (75 out of 100 or ¾).

To calculate a percentage, divide the number of items or patients in the category by the total number in the group and multiply by 100.

**EXAMPLE**

Data were collected on 80 patients referred for heart transplantation. The researcher wanted to compare their ages. The data for age were put in "decade bands" and are shown in *Table 1*.

Table 1. Ages of 80 patients referred for heart transplantation

| Years[a] | Frequency[b] | Percentage[c] |
|---|---|---|
| 0–9 | 2 | 2.5 |
| 10–19 | 5 | 6.25 |
| 20–29 | 6 | 7.5 |
| 30–39 | 14 | 17.5 |
| 40–49 | 21 | 26.25 |
| 50–59 | 20 | 25 |
| ≥ 60 | 12 | 15 |
| Total | 80 | 100 |

[a] Years = decade bands;

[b] Frequency = number of patients referred;

[c] Percentage = percentage of patients in each decade band. For example, in the 30–39 age band there were 14 patients and we know the ages of 80 patients, so $\frac{14}{80} \times 100 = 17.5\%$.

## Watch out for . . .

Some papers refer to "proportions" rather than percentages. A proportion is the number of items or patients in the category divided by the total number in the group, but unlike a percentage it is not then multiplied by 100.

Authors can use percentages to hide the true size of the data. To say that 50% of a sample has a certain condition when there are only four people in the sample is clearly not providing the same level of information as 50% of a sample based on 400 people. So, percentages should be used as an additional help for the reader rather than replacing the actual data.

## Ch 4  MEAN

Otherwise known as an "arithmetic mean" or "average".

### How important is it?

 A mean appeared in 70% of papers surveyed, so it is important to have an understanding of how it is calculated.

### How easy is it to understand?

One of the simplest statistical concepts to grasp. However, in most groups that we have taught there has been at least one person who admits not knowing how to calculate the mean, so we do not apologize for including it here.

### When is it used?

It is used when the spread of the data is fairly similar on each side of the mid point, for example when the data are "normally distributed".

The "normal distribution" (sometimes called the "Gaussian distribution") is referred to a lot in statistics. It's the symmetrical, bell-shaped distribution of data shown in *Fig. 1*.

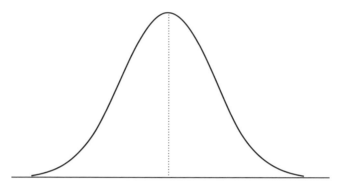

**Fig. 1.** The normal distribution. The dotted line shows the mean of the data.

### What does it mean?

The mean is the sum of all the values, divided by the number of values.

---

**EXAMPLE**

Five women in a study on lipid-lowering agents are aged 55, 59, 52, 58 and 56 years.

Add these ages together:

$55 + 59 + 52 + 58 + 56 = 280$

Now divide by the number of women:

$$\frac{280}{5} = 56$$

So the mean age is 56 years.

---

### Watch out for...

If a value (or a number of values) is a lot smaller or larger than the others, "skewing" the data, the mean will then not give a good picture of the typical value.

For example, if there is a sixth patient aged 92 in the study then the mean age would be 62, even though only one woman is over 60 years old. In this case, the "median" may be a more suitable mid-point to use (see *Chapter 5*).

A common multiple choice question is to ask the difference between mean, median (see *Chapter 5*) and mode (see *Chapter 6*) – make sure that you do not get confused between them.

## Ch 5 MEDIAN

Sometimes known as the "midpoint".

## How important is it?

✪✪✪✪     It is given in almost half of mainstream papers.

## How easy is it to understand?

👍👍👍👍👍     Even easier than the mean!

## When is it used?

It is used to represent the average when the data are not symmetrical, for instance the "skewed" distribution in *Fig. 2*. Compare the shape of the graph with the normal distribution shown in *Fig. 1*.

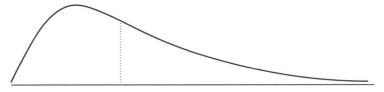

**Fig. 2.** A skewed distribution. The dotted line shows the median.

## What does it mean?

It is the point which has half the values above, and half below.

**EXAMPLE**

Using the first example from *Chapter 4*, putting the five patients in age order gives 52, 55, 56, 58 and 59. The median age is 56, the same as the mean – half the women are older, half are younger.

However, in the second example with six patients aged 52, 55, 56, 58, 59 and 92 years, there are two "middle" ages, 56 and 58. The median is half-way between these, i.e. 57 years. This gives a better idea of the mid-point of these skewed data than the mean of 62.

## Watch out for...

The median may be given with its inter-quartile range (IQR). The 1$^{st}$ quartile point has the ¼ of the data below it, the 3$^{rd}$ quartile point has the ¾ of the sample below it, so the IQR contains the middle ½ of the sample. This can be shown in a "box and whisker" plot.

**EXAMPLE**

A dietician measured the energy intake over 24 hours of 50 patients on a variety of wards. One ward had two patients that were "nil by mouth". The median was 12.2 megajoules, IQR 9.9 to 13.6. The lowest intake was 0, the highest was 16.7. This distribution is represented by the box and whisker plot in *Fig. 3*.

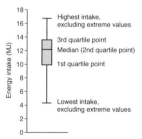

**Fig. 3.** Box and whisker plot of energy intake of 50 patients over 24 hours. The ends of the whiskers represent the maximum and minimum values, excluding extreme results like those of the two "nil by mouth" patients.

## Ch 6 MODE

### How important is it?

✪         Rarely quoted in papers and of limited value.

### How easy is it to understand?

👍👍👍👍👍    An easy concept.

### When is it used?

It is used when we need a label for the most frequently occurring event.

### What does it mean?

The mode is the most common of a set of events.

---

**EXAMPLE**

An eye clinic sister noted the eye colour of 100 consecutive patients. The results are shown in *Fig. 4*.

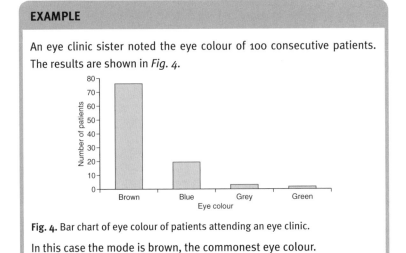

**Fig. 4.** Bar chart of eye colour of patients attending an eye clinic.

In this case the mode is brown, the commonest eye colour.

You may see reference to a "bi-modal distribution". Generally when this is mentioned in papers it is as a concept rather than from calculating the actual values, e.g. "The data appear to follow a bi-modal distribution". See *Fig. 5* for an example of where there are two "peaks" to the data, i.e. a bi-modal distribution.

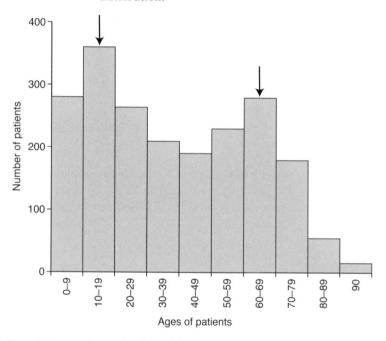

**Fig. 5.** Histogram of ages of patients with asthma in a practice.

The arrows point to the modes at ages 10–19 and 60–69.

Bi-modal data may suggest that two populations are present that are mixed together, so an average is not a suitable measure for the distribution.

# Ch 7   STANDARD DEVIATION

## How important is it?

✪✪✪✪✪   Quoted in two-thirds of papers, it is used as the basis of a number of statistical calculations.

## How easy is it to understand?

   It is not an intuitive concept.

## When is it used?

Standard deviation (SD) is used for data which are "normally distributed" (see *Chapter 4*), to provide information on how much the data vary around their mean.

## What does it mean?

SD indicates how much a set of values is spread around the average.

A range of one SD above and below the mean (abbreviated to ± 1 SD) includes 68.2% of the values.

± 2 SD includes 95.4% of the data.

± 3 SD includes 99.7%.

**EXAMPLE**

Let us say that a group of patients enrolling for a trial had a normal distribution for weight. The mean weight of the patients was 80 kg. For this group, the SD was calculated to be 5 kg.

1 SD below the average is 80 – 5 = 75 kg.

1 SD above the average is 80 + 5 = 85 kg.

± 1 SD will include 68.2% of the subjects, so 68.2% of patients will weigh between 75 and 85 kg.

95.4% will weigh between 70 and 90 kg (± 2 SD).

99.7% of patients will weigh between 65 and 95 kg (± 3 SD).

See how this relates to the graph of the data in *Fig. 6.*

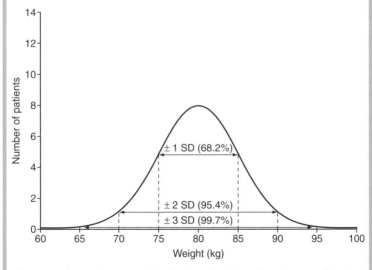

**Fig. 6.** Graph showing normal distribution of weights of patients enrolling in a trial with mean 80 kg, SD 5 kg.

If we have two sets of data with the same mean but different SDs, then the data set with the smaller SD has a narrower spread than the data set with the larger SD.

For example, if another group of patients enrolling for the trial has the same mean weight of 80 kg but an SD of only 3, ± 1 SD will include 68.2% of the subjects, so 68.2% of patients will weigh between 77 and 83 kg (*Fig. 7*). Compare this with the example above.

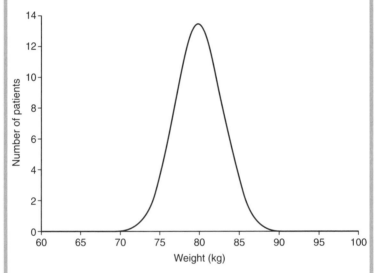

**Fig. 7.** Graph showing normal distribution of weights of patients enrolling in a trial with mean 80 kg, SD 3 kg.

## Watch out for...

SD should only be used when the data have a normal distribution. However, means and SDs are often wrongly used for data which are not normally distributed.

A simple check for a normal distribution is to see if 2 SDs away from the mean are still within the possible range for the variable. For example, if we have some length of hospital stay data with a mean stay of 10 days and a SD of 8 days then:

mean – (2 × SD) = 10 – (2 × 8) = 10 – 16 = –6 days.

This is clearly an impossible value for length of stay, so the data cannot be normally distributed. The mean and SDs are therefore not appropriate measures to use.

Good news – it is not necessary to know how to calculate the SD.

It *is* worth learning the figures above off by heart, so a reminder –

± 1 SD includes 68.2% of the data

± 2 SD includes 95.4%,

± 3 SD includes 99.7%.

Keeping the "normal distribution" curve in *Fig.* 6 in mind may help.

Examiners may ask what percentages of subjects are included in 1, 2 or 3 SDs from the mean. Again, try to memorize those percentages.

### How important are they?

✪✪✪✪✪          Important – given in four out of every five papers.

### How easy are they to understand?

👍 👍          A difficult concept, but one where a small amount of understanding will get you by without having to worry about the details.

### When is it used?

Confidence intervals (CI) are typically used when, instead of simply wanting the mean value of a sample, we want a range that is likely to contain the true population value.

This "true value" is another tough concept – it is the mean value that we would get if we had data for the whole population.

### What does it mean?

Statisticians can calculate a range (interval) in which we can be fairly sure (confident) that the "true value" lies.

For example, we may be interested in blood pressure (BP) reduction with antihypertensive treatment. From a sample of treated patients we can work out the mean change in BP.

However, this will only be the mean for our particular sample. If we took another group of patients we would not expect to get exactly the same value, because chance can also affect the change in BP.

The CI gives the range in which the true value (i.e. the mean change in BP if we treated an infinite number of patients) is likely to be.

## EXAMPLES

The average systolic BP before treatment in study A, of a group of 100 hypertensive patients, was 170 mmHg. After treatment with the new drug the mean BP dropped by 20 mmHg.

If the 95% CI is 15–25, this means we can be 95% confident that the true effect of treatment is to lower the BP by 15–25 mmHg.

In study B 50 patients were treated with the same drug, also reducing their mean BP by 20 mmHg, but with a wider 95% CI of -5 to +45. This CI includes zero (no change). This means there is more than a 5% chance that there was no true change in BP, and that the drug was actually ineffective.

## Watch out for...

The size of a CI is related to the size of the sample and the variability of the individual results. Larger studies usually have a narrower CI.

Where a few interventions, outcomes or studies are given it is difficult to visualize a long list of means and CIs. Some papers will show a chart to make it easier.

For example, "meta-analysis" is a technique for bringing together results from a number of similar studies to give one overall estimate of effect. Many meta-analyses compare the treatment effects from those studies by showing the mean changes and 95% CIs in a chart. An example is given in *Fig. 8*.

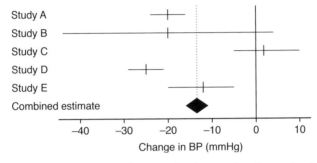

**Fig. 8.** Plot of 5 studies of a new antihypertensive drug. See how the results of studies A and B above are shown by the top two lines, i.e. a 20 mmHg reduction in BP, 95% CI 15–25 for study A and a 20 mmHg reduction, 95% CI -5 to +45 for study B.

The long vertical line represents the point showing "no change" or "no effect".

The statistician has combined the results of all five studies and calculated that the overall mean reduction in BP is 14 mmHg, CI 12–16. This is shown by the "combined estimate" diamond and the dotted line. See how combining a number of studies reduces the CI, giving a more accurate estimate of the true treatment effect.

The chart shown in *Fig. 8* is called a "Forest plot" or, more colloquially, a "blobbogram".

**Standard deviation and confidence intervals – what is the difference?** Standard deviation tells us about the variability (spread) in a sample.

The CI tells us the range in which the true value (the mean if the sample were infinitely large) is likely to be.

An exam question may give a chart similar to that in *Fig. 8* and ask you to summarize the findings. Consider:

- Which study showed the greatest change?

- Did all the studies show change in favour of the intervention?

- Does the combined estimate exclude no difference between the treatments?

In the example above, study D showed the greatest change, with a mean BP drop of 25 mmHg.

Study C resulted in a mean increase in BP, though with a wider CI. This CI could be due to a low number of patients in the study. Note that the CI crosses the line of "no effect".

The combined estimate of the mean BP reduction is 14 mmHg, 95% CI 12–16. This tells us that the "true value" for the reduction in BP is likely to be between 12 and 16 mmHg, and this excludes "no difference" between the treatments.

## Ch 9  *P* VALUES

### How important is it?

✪✪✪✪  A really important concept, *P* values are given in more than two-thirds of papers.

### How easy is it to understand?

👍👍👍  Not easy, but worth persevering as it is used so frequently.

It is not essential to know how the *P* value is derived – just to be able to interpret the result.

### When is it used?

The *P* (probability) value is used when we wish to see how likely it is that a hypothesis is true. The hypothesis is usually that there is *no* difference between two treatments, known as the "null hypothesis".

### What does it mean?

The *P* value gives the probability of any observed difference having happened by chance.

$P = 0.5$ means that the probability of a difference this large or larger having happened by chance is 0.5 in 1, or 50:50.

$P = 0.05$ means that the probability of a difference this large or larger having happened by chance is 0.05 in 1, i.e. 1 in 20.

It is the figure frequently quoted as being "statistically significant", i.e. unlikely to have happened by chance and therefore important. However, this is an arbitrary figure.

If we look at 20 studies, even if none of the treatments really work, one of the studies is likely to have a *P* value of 0.05 and so appear significant!

The lower the *P* value, the less likely it is that the difference happened by chance and so the higher the significance of the finding.

*P* = 0.01 is often considered to be "highly significant". It means that a difference of this size or larger will only have happened by chance 1 in 100 times. This is unlikely, but still possible.

*P* = 0.001 means that a difference of this size or larger will have happened by chance 1 in 1000 times, even less likely, but still just possible. It is usually considered to be "very highly significant".

**EXAMPLES**

Out of 50 new babies on average 25 will be girls, sometimes more, sometimes less.

Say there is a new fertility treatment and we want to know whether it affects the chance of having a boy or a girl. Therefore we set up a "null hypothesis" – that the treatment *does not* alter the chance of having a girl. Out of the first 50 babies resulting from the treatment, 15 are girls. We then need to know the probability that this just happened by chance, i.e. did this happen by chance or has the treatment had an effect on the sex of the babies?

The *P* value gives the probability that the null hypothesis is true.

The *P* value in this example is 0.007. Do not worry about how it was calculated, concentrate on what it means. It means the result would only have happened by chance in 0.007 in 1 (or 1 in 140) times if the treatment did not actually affect the sex of the baby. This is highly unlikely, so we can reject our hypothesis and conclude that the treatment probably *does* alter the chance of having a girl.

***Try another example:*** Patients with minor illnesses were randomized to see either Dr Smith or Dr Jones. Dr Smith ended up seeing 176 patients in the study whereas Dr Jones saw 200 patients (*Table 2*).

**Table 2.** Number of patients with minor illnesses seen by two GPs

| | Dr Jones (n=200)[a] | Dr Smith (n=176) | P value | i.e. could have happened by chance |
|---|---|---|---|---|
| Patients satisfied with consultation (%) | 186 (93) | 168 (95) | 0.38 | About four times in 10 – possible |
| Mean (SD) consultation length (minutes) | 16 (3.1) | 6 (2.8) | <0.001 | < One time in 1000 – very unlikely |
| Patients getting a prescription (%) | 65 (33) | 67 (38) | 0.28 | About three times in 10 – possible |
| Mean (SD) number of days off work | 3.58 (1.3) | 3.61 (1.3) | 0.82 | About eight times in 10 – probable |
| Patients needing a follow-up appointment (%) | 68 (34) | 78 (44) | 0.044 | Only one time in 23 – fairly unlikely |

[a] n=200 means that the total number of patients seen by Dr Jones was 200.

## Watch out for...

The "null hypothesis" is a concept that underlies this and other statistical tests.

The test method assumes (hypothesizes) that there is *no* (null) difference between the groups. The result of the test either supports or rejects that hypothesis.

The null hypothesis is generally the opposite of what we are actually interested in finding out. If we are interested if there is a difference between two treatments then the null hypothesis would be that there is no difference and we would try to disprove this.

Try not to confuse statistical significance with clinical relevance. If a study is too small, the results are unlikely to be statistically significant even if the intervention actually works. Conversely a large study may find a statistically significant difference that is too small to have any clinical relevance.

You may be given a set of *P* values and asked to interpret them. Remember that $P = 0.05$ is usually classed as "significant", $P = 0.01$ as "highly significant" and $P = 0.001$ as "very highly significant".

In the example above, only two of the sets of data showed a significant difference between the two GPs. Dr Smith's consultations were very highly significantly shorter than those of Dr Jones. Dr Smith's follow-up rate was significantly higher than that of Dr Jones.

# Ch 10  *t* TESTS AND OTHER PARAMETRIC TESTS

## How important are they?

✪✪✪✪      Used in one in three papers, they are an important aspect of medical statistics.

## How easy are they to understand?

👍      The details of the tests themselves are difficult to understand.

Thankfully you do not need to know them. Just look for the *P* value (see *Chapter 9*) to see how significant the result is. Remember, the smaller the *P* value, the smaller the chance that the "null hypothesis" is true.

## When are they used?

Parametric statistics are used to compare samples of "normally distributed" data (see *Chapter 4*). If the data do *not* follow a normal distribution, these tests should not be used.

## What do they mean?

A parametric test is any test which requires the data to follow a specific distribution, usually a normal distribution. Common parametric tests you will come across are the ANOVA and the *t* test.

**Analysis of variance (ANOVA).** This is a group of statistical techniques used to compare the means of two or more samples to see whether they come from the same population – the "null hypothesis". These techniques can also allow for independent variables which may have an effect on the outcome.

Again, check out the *P* value.

***t* test (also known as Student's t).** *t* tests are typically used to compare just two samples. They test the probability that the samples come from a population with the same mean value.

---

### EXAMPLE

Two hundred adults seeing an asthma nurse specialist were randomly assigned to either a new type of bronchodilator or placebo.

After 3 months the peak flow rates in the treatment group had increased by a mean of 96 l/min (SD 58), and in the placebo group by 70 l/min (SD 52). The null hypothesis is that there is <u>no</u> difference between the bronchodilator and the placebo.

The *t* statistic is 11.14, resulting in a *P* value of 0.001. It is therefore very unlikely (1 in 1000 chance) that the null hypothesis is correct so we reject the hypothesis and conclude that the new bronchodilator is significantly better than the placebo.

---

## Watch out for...

Parametric tests should only be used when the data follow a "normal" distribution. You may find reference to the "Kolmogorov Smirnov" test. This tests the hypothesis that the collected data are from a normal distribution and therefore assesses whether parametric statistics can be used.

Sometimes authors will say that they have "transformed" data and then analyzed them with a parametric test. This is quite legitimate – it is not cheating! For example, a skewed distribution might become normally distributed if the logarithm of the values is used.

# Ch 11 MANN–WHITNEY AND OTHER NON-PARAMETRIC TESTS

## How important are they?

✪✪             Used in one in ten papers.

## How easy are they to understand?

👍             Non-parametric testing is difficult to understand.

However, you do not need to know the details of the tests. Look out for the *P* value (see *Chapter 9*) to see how significant the results are. Remember, the smaller the *P* value, the smaller the chance that the "null hypothesis" is true.

## When are they used?

Non-parametric statistics are used when the data are *not* normally distributed and so are not appropriate for "parametric" tests.

## What do they mean?

Rather than comparing the values of the raw data, statisticians "rank" the data and compare the ranks.

**EXAMPLE**

*Mann–Whitney U test.* A GP introduced a nurse triage system into her practice. She was interested in finding out whether the age of the patients attending for triage appointments was different to that of patients who made emergency appointments with the GP.

The triage nurse saw 646 patients and the GP saw 532. The median age of the triage nurse's patients was 50 years (1st quartile 40 years, 3rd quartile 54), for the GP it was 46 (22, 58). Note how the quartiles show an uneven distribution around the median, so the data cannot be normally distributed and a non-parametric test is appropriate. The graph in *Fig. 9* shows the ages of the patients seen by the nurse and confirms a skewed, rather than normal, distribution.

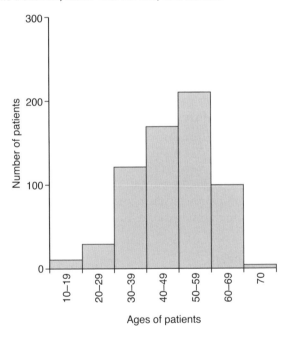

**Fig. 9.** Histogram of ages of patients seen by triage nurse.

The statistician used a "Mann–Whitney U test" to test the hypothesis that there is no difference between the ages of the two groups. This gave a U value of 133 200 with a $P$ value of < 0.001. Ignore the actual U value but concentrate on the $P$ value, which in this case suggests that the triage nurse's patients were very highly significantly older than those who saw the GP.

Note that this statistic does not state the size of that difference, only that there is very unlikely to be no difference.

## Watch out for...

The "Wilcoxon signed rank test", "Kruskal Wallis" and "Friedman" tests are other non-parametric tests. Do not be put off by the names – go straight to the $P$ value.

# Ch 12 CHI-SQUARED TEST

Usually written as $\chi^2$ (for the test) or $X^2$ (for its value), chi is pronounced as in sky without the s.

## How important is it?

✪✪✪✪  A frequently used test of significance, given in a quarter of papers.

## How easy is it to understand?

  Do not try to understand the $X^2$ value, just look at whether or not the result is significant.

## When is it used?

It is a measure of the difference between actual and expected frequencies.

## What does it mean?

The "expected frequency" is the frequency we would see if the null hypothesis were true. If the observed and the expected frequencies were the same, the $X^2$ value would be zero.

The larger the actual difference between the sets of results, the greater the $X^2$ value. However, it is difficult to interpret the $X^2$ value by itself as it depends on the number of factors studied.

Statisticians make it easier for you by giving the *P* value (see *Chapter 9*), giving you the likelihood there is no real difference between the groups.

So, do not worry about the actual value of $X^2$ but look at its *P* value.

---

**EXAMPLE**

Patients with bronchopneumonia were treated with either amoxicillin or erythromycin. The results are shown in *Table 3*.

**Table 3.** Comparison of effect of treatment of bronchopneumonia with amoxicillin or erythromycin

|  | Type of antibiotic given | | | | | |
|---|---|---|---|---|---|---|
|  | Amoxicillin | | Erythromycin | | Total | |
| Improvement at 5 days | 144 | (60%) | 160 | (67%) | 304 | (63%) |
| No improvement at 5 days | 96 | (40%) | 80 | (33%) | 176 | (37%) |
| Total | 240 | (100%) | 240 | (100%) | 480 | (100%) |
|  | $X^2 = 2.3$; $P = 0.13$ | | | | | |

A table like this is known as a "contingency table" or "two-way table".

First, look at the table to get an idea of the differences between the effects of the two treatments, then look for the chi-squared test result and its *P* value.

Remember, do not worry about the $X^2$ value itself, but see whether it is significant. In this case *P* is 0.13, so the difference in treatments is not statistically significant.

---

## Watch out for...

Some papers will also give the "degrees of freedom" (df), for example $X^2 = 2.3$; df 1; $P = 0.13$. See *Glossary* for an explanation. This is used with the $X^2$ value to work out the *P* value.

***Other tests you may find.*** Instead of the $\chi^2$ test, "Fisher's exact test" is sometimes used to analyze contingency tables. Fisher's test is the best choice as it always gives the exact *P* value, particularly where the numbers are small.

The $\chi^2$ test is simpler for statisticians to calculate but gives only an approximate $P$ value and is inappropriate for small samples. Statisticians may apply "Yates' continuity correction" or other adjustments to the $\chi^2$ test to improve the accuracy of the $P$ value.

The "Mantel Haenszel test" is an extension of the $\chi^2$ test that is used to compare several two-way tables.

# Ch 13 RISK RATIO

Often referred to as "relative risk".

## How important is it?

✪✪✪     Used in one in five papers.

## How easy is it to understand?

 Risk is a relatively intuitive concept that we encounter every day, but interpretation of risk (especially low risk) is often inconsistent. The risk of death while travelling to the shops to buy a lottery ticket can be higher than the risk of winning the jackpot!

## When is it used?

Relative risk is used in "cohort studies", prospective studies that follow a group (cohort) over a period of time and investigate the effect of a treatment or risk factor.

## What does it mean?

First, risk itself. *Risk* is the probability that an event will happen. It is calculated by dividing the number of events by the number of people at risk.

One boy is born for every two births, so the probability (risk) of giving birth to a boy is

½ = 0.5

If one in every 100 patients suffers a side-effect from a treatment, the risk is

$\frac{1}{100} = 0.01$

Compare this with odds (*Chapter 14*).

Now, risk *ratios*. These are calculated by dividing the risk in the treated or exposed group by the risk in the control or unexposed group.

A risk ratio of one indicates no difference in risk between the groups.

If the risk ratio of an event is >1, the rate of that event is increased compared to controls.

If <1, the rate of that event is reduced.

Risk ratios are frequently given with their 95% CIs: if the CI for a risk ratio *does not* include one (no difference in risk), it is statistically significant.

**EXAMPLE**

Cohorts of 1000 regular football players and 1000 non-footballers were followed to see if playing football was significant in the injuries that they received.

After 1 year of follow-up there had been 12 broken legs in the football players and only 4 in the non-footballers.

The *risk* of a footballer breaking a leg was therefore 12/1000 or 0.012. The risk of a non-footballer breaking a leg was 4/1000 or 0.004.

The risk *ratio* of breaking a leg was therefore 0.012/0.004 which equals 3. The 95% CI was calculated to be 0.97 to 9.41. As the CI includes the value 1 we cannot exclude the possibility that there was no difference in the risk of footballers and non-footballers breaking a leg. However, given these results further research would clearly be warranted.

# Ch 14 ODDS RATIO

## How important is it?

✪✪✪✪          Used in a third of papers.

## How easy is it to understand?

          Odds are difficult to understand. Just aim to understand what the ratio means.

## When is it used?

Used by epidemiologists in studies looking for factors which do harm, it is a way of comparing patients who already have a certain condition (cases) with patients who do not (controls) – a "case–control study".

## What does it mean?

First, *odds*. Odds are calculated by dividing the number of times an event happens by the number of times it does not happen.

One boy is born for every two births, so the odds of giving birth to a boy are

$1:1$ (or 50:50) = $\frac{1}{1}$ = 1

If one in every 100 patients suffers a side-effect from a treatment, the odds are

$1:99 = \frac{1}{99} = 0.0101$

Compare this with risk (see *Chapter 13*).

Next, odds *ratios*. They are calculated by dividing the odds of having been exposed to a risk factor by the odds in the control group.

An odds ratio of 1 indicates no difference in risk between the groups, i.e. the odds in each group are the same.

If the odds ratio of an event is >1, the rate of that event is increased in patients who have been exposed to the risk factor.

If <1, the rate of that event is reduced.

Odds ratios are frequently given with their 95% CI: if the CI for an odds ratio *does not* include 1 (no difference in odds), it is statistically significant.

## EXAMPLES

A group of 100 patients with knee injuries, "cases", was matched for age and sex to 100 patients who did not have injured knees, "controls".

In the cases, 40 skied and 60 did not, giving the *odds* of being a skier for this group of 40:60 or 0.66.

In the controls, 20 patients skied and 80 did not, giving the odds of being a skier for the control group of 20:80 or 0.25.

We can therefore calculate the odds *ratio* as 0.66/0.25 = 2.64. The 95% CI is 1.41 to 5.02.

If you cannot follow the maths, do not worry! The odds ratio means that the odds for a case being a skier are 2.64 times that for a control being a skier, and as the CI does not include 1 (no difference in risk) this is statistically significant. Therefore, we can conclude that patients with these knee injuries are significantly more likely to be skiers than those without knee injuries.

## Watch out for...

Authors may give the percentage *change* in the odds ratio rather than the odds ratio itself. In the example above, the odds ratio of 2.64 means the same as a 164% increase in the odds of patients with injured knees being skiers.

Odds ratios are often interpreted by the reader in the same way as risk ratios. This is reasonable when the odds are low, but for common events the odds and the risks (and therefore their ratios) will give very different values. For example, the odds of giving birth to a boy are 1, whereas the risk is 0.5. However, in the side-effect example given above the odds are 0.0101, a similar value to the risk of 0.01. For this reason, if you are looking at a case–control study, check that the authors have used odds ratios rather than risk ratios.

## Ch 15 RISK REDUCTION AND NUMBERS NEEDED TO TREAT

### How important are they?

✪✪✪      Although only quoted in less than 5% of papers, they are helpful in trying to work out how worthwhile a treatment is in clinical practice.

### How easy are they to understand?

👍👍👍👍👍    "Relative risk reduction" (RRR) and "absolute risk reduction" (ARR) need some concentration. "Numbers needed to treat" (NNT) are pretty intuitive, useful and not too difficult to work out for yourself.

### When are they used?

They are used when an author wants to know how often a treatment works, rather than just whether it works.

### What do they mean?

ARR is the difference between the event rate in the intervention group and that in the control group. It is usually given as a percentage.

NNT is the number of patients who need to be treated for one to get benefit. It is 100 divided by the ARR, i.e. $NNT = \dfrac{100}{ARR}$

RRR is the proportion by which the intervention reduces the event rate. It is calculated by dividing the ARR by the control event rate.

## EXAMPLES

One hundred women with vaginal candida were given an oral antifungal, 100 were given placebo. They were reviewed 3 days later. The results are given in *Table 4*.

**Table 4.** Results of placebo-controlled trial of oral antifungal agent

| Given antifungal | | Given placebo | |
|---|---|---|---|
| Improved | No improvement | Improved | No improvement |
| 80 | 20 | 60 | 40 |

ARR = improvement rate in the intervention group – improvement rate in the control group = 80% – 60% = 20%

$$NNT = \frac{100}{ARR} = \frac{100}{20} = 5$$

So five women have to be treated for one to get benefit.

The incidence of candidiasis was reduced from 40% with placebo to 20% with treatment, so

$$RRR = \frac{ARR}{Control\ (placebo)\ event\ rate} = \frac{20}{40} = 0.5,\ \text{which is 50\%.}$$

Thus, the RRR is 50%.

In another trial, young men were treated with an expensive lipid-lowering agent. Five years later the death rate from ischaemic heart disease (IHD) was recorded. See *Table 5* for the results.

**Table 5.** Results of placebo-controlled trial of Cleverstatin

| Given Cleverstatin | | Given placebo | |
|---|---|---|---|
| Survived | Died | Survived | Died |
| 998 (99.8%) | 2 (0.2%) | 997 (99.7%) | 3 (0.3%) |

ARR = improvement rate in the intervention group – improvement rate in the control group = 99.8% – 99.7% = 0.1%

$$NNT = \frac{100}{ARR} = \frac{100}{0.1} = 1000$$

So 1000 men have to be treated for 5 years for one to survive who would otherwise have died.

The incidence of death from IHD is reduced from 0.3% with placebo to 0.2% with treatment, so

$$RRR = \frac{ARR}{\text{Control (placebo) event rate}} = \frac{0.3-0.2}{0.3} = \frac{0.1}{0.3} = 0.333,$$
which is 33.3%

Thus, the RRR is 33%.

The RRR and NNT from the same study can have opposing effects on prescribing habits. The RRR of 33% in this example sounds fantastic. However, thinking of it in terms of an NNT of 1000 might sound less attractive: for every life saved, 999 patients had unnecessary treatment for 5 years.

## Watch out for...

Usually the necessary percentages are given in the abstract of the paper. Calculating the ARR is easy: subtract the percentage that improved without treatment from the percentage that improved with treatment.

Again, dividing that figure into 100 gives the NNT.

With an NNT you need to know:

(a) What treatment?

- What are the side-effects?

- What is the cost?

(b) For how long?

(c) To achieve what?

- How serious is the event you are trying to avoid?

- How easy is it to treat if it happens?

For treatments, the lower the NNT the better – but look at the context.

(a) NNT of 10 for treating a sore throat with expensive blundamycin

- not attractive

(b) NNT of 10 for prevention of death from leukaemia with a non-toxic chemotherapy agent

- worthwhile

Expect NNTs for prophylaxis to be much larger. For example, an immunization may have an NNT in the thousands but still be well worthwhile.

**Numbers needed to harm** (NNH) may also be important.

$$NNH = \frac{100}{(\% \text{ on treatment that had SEs}) + (\% \text{ not on treatment that had SEs})}$$

In the example above, 6% of those on cleverstatin had peptic ulceration as opposed to 1% of those on placebo.

$$NNH = \frac{100}{6-1} = \frac{100}{5} = 20$$

i.e. for every 20 patients treated, one peptic ulcer was caused.

You may see ARR and RRR given as a proportion instead of a percentage. So, an ARR of 20% is the same as an ARR of 0.2. Where the ARR is given as a proportion rather than as a percentage, the equation to calculate the NNT is this:

$$NNT = \frac{1}{ARR}$$

Be prepared to calculate RRR, ARR and NNT from a set of results. You may find that it helps to draw a simple table like *Table 5* and work from there.

## Ch 16 CORRELATION

### How important is it?

  Only used in 15% of medical papers.

### How easy is it to understand?

### When is it used?

Where there is a linear relationship between two variables there is said to be a correlation between them. Examples are height and weight in children, or socio-economic class and mortality.

The *strength* of that relationship is given by the "correlation coefficient".

### What does it mean?

The correlation coefficient is usually denoted by the letter "$r$", for example $r = 0.8$.

A *positive* correlation coefficient means that as one variable is increasing, the value for the other variable is also increasing – the line on the graph slopes up from left to right. Height and weight have a positive correlation: children get heavier as they grow taller.

A *negative* correlation coefficient means that as the value of one variable goes up, the value for the other variable goes down – the graph slopes down from left to right. Higher socio-economic class is associated with a lower mortality, giving a negative correlation between the two variables.

If there is a perfect relationship between the two variables then $r = 1$ (if a positive correlation) or $r = -1$ (if a negative correlation).

If there is no correlation at all (the points on the graph are completely randomly scattered) then $r = 0$.

The following is a good rule of thumb when considering the size of a correlation:

$r = 0{-}0.2$ : very low and probably meaningless.

$r = 0.2{-}0.4$ : a low correlation that might warrant further investigation.

$r = 0.4{-}0.6$ : a reasonable correlation.

$r = 0.6{-}0.8$ : a high correlation.

$r = 0.8{-}1.0$ : a very high correlation. Possibly too high! Check for errors or other reasons for such a high correlation.

This guide also applies to negative correlations.

## EXAMPLES

A nurse wanted to be able to predict the laboratory HbA1c result (a measure of blood glucose control) from the fasting blood glucoses which she measured in her clinic. On 12 consecutive diabetic patients she noted the fasting glucose and simultaneously drew blood for HbA1c. She compared the pairs of measurements and drew the graph in *Fig. 10*.

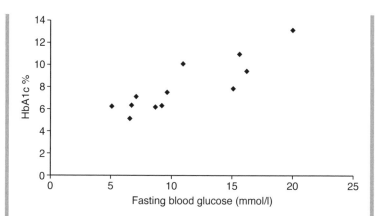

**Fig. 10.** Plot of fasting glucose and HbA1c in 12 patients with diabetes. For these results $r = 0.88$, showing a very high correlation.

A graph like this is known as a "scatter plot".

An occupational therapist developed a scale for measuring physical activity and wondered how much it correlated to Body Mass Index (BMI) in 12 of her adult patients. *Fig. 11* shows how they related.

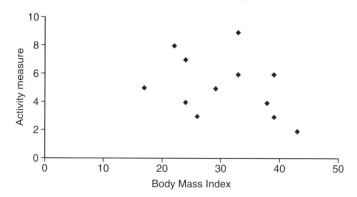

**Fig. 11.** BMI and activity measure in 12 adult patients.

In this example, $r = -0.34$, indicating a low correlation. The fact that the $r$ value is negative shows that the correlation is negative, indicating that patients with a higher level of physical activity tended to have a lower BMI.

## Watch out for...

Correlation tells us how strong the association between the variables is, but does not tell us about cause and effect in that relationship.

The "Pearson correlation coefficient", Pearson's $r$, is used if the values are sampled from "normal" populations (see *Chapter 4*). Otherwise the "Spearman rank correlation coefficient" is used. However, the interpretation of the two is the same.

Where the author shows the graph, you can get a good idea from the scatter as to how strong the relationship is without needing to know the $r$ value.

The statistical significance of a correlation only states how reliable that $r$ value is, it does not indicate its clinical importance. If a study is sufficiently large, even a small clinically unimportant correlation will be highly significant. So, we need to consider the size of the correlation.

A correlation coefficient may also be given with its confidence interval (see *Chapter 8*).

$R^2$ is sometimes given. As it is the square of the $r$ value, and squares are always positive, you cannot use it to tell whether the graph slopes up or down.

What it *does* tell you is how much of the variation in one value is related to the variation in the other value.

In *Fig. 10*, $r = 0.88$. $R^2 = 0.88 \times 0.88 = 0.77$. This means that 77% of the variation in HbA1c is related to the variation in fasting glucose.

Again, the closer the $R^2$ value is to 1, the higher the correlation.

It is very easy for authors to compare a large number of variables using correlation and only present the ones that happen to be significant. So, check to make sure there is a plausible explanation for any significant correlations.

Also bear in mind that a correlation only tells us about linear (straight line) relationships between variables. Two variables may be strongly related but not in a straight line, giving a low $r$ value.

## Ch 17 REGRESSION

### How important is it?

✪✪        Regression analysis is used in around 20% of papers.

### How easy is it to understand?

     The idea of trying to fit a line through a set of points to make the line as representative as possible is relatively straightforward. However, the mathematics involved in fitting regression models are more difficult to understand.

### When is it used?

Regression analysis is used to find how one set of data relates to another.

This can be particularly helpful where we want to use one measure as a substitute for another – for example, a near-patient test to avoid the need for a lab test.

### What does it mean?

A "regression line" is the line that fits best through the data points on a graph. This is often calculated using a technique called "least squares".

The "regression coefficient" gives the gradient of the graph, in that it gives the change in value of one outcome, per unit change in the other.

**EXAMPLE**

Consider the graph shown in *Fig. 10* (see *Chapter 16*). A statistician calculated the line that gave the "best fit" through the scatter of points, shown in *Fig. 12*.

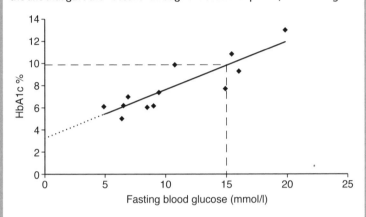

**Fig. 12.** Plot with linear regression line of fasting glucose and HbA1c in 12 patients with diabetes.

The line is called a "regression line".

To predict the HbA1c for a given blood glucose a nurse could simply plot it on the graph, as here where a fasting glucose of 15 predicts an HbA1c of approximately 9.9%.

This can also be done mathematically. The gradient and position of the regression line can be represented by the "regression equation":

HbA1c = 3.2 + (0.45 × blood glucose).

The 0.45 figure gives the *gradient* of the graph and is called the "regression coefficient".

The "regression constant" that gives the *position* of the line on the graph is 3.2: it is the point where the line crosses the vertical axis.

Try this with a glucose of 15:

HbA1c = 3.2 + (0.45 x 15) = 3.2 + 6.75 = 9.95%

This regression equation can be applied to any regression line. It is represented by:

$y = a + bx$

To predict the value y (value on the vertical axis of the graph) from the value x (on the horizontal axis), b is the regression coefficient and a is the constant.

## Other values sometimes given with regression

You may see other values quoted. The regression coefficient and constant can be given with their "standard errors". These indicate the accuracy that can be given to the calculations. Do not worry about the actual value of these but look at their $P$ values. The lower the $P$ value, the greater the significance.

The $R^2$ value may also be given. This represents the amount of the variation in the data that is explained by the regression. In our example the $R^2$ value is 0.77. This is stating that 77% of the variation in the HbA1c result is accounted for by variation in the blood glucose.

## Other types of regression

The example above is a "linear regression", as the line that best fits the points is straight.

Other forms of regression include:

*Logistic regression.* This is used where each case in the sample can only belong to one of two groups (e.g. having disease or not) with the outcome as the probability that a case belongs to one group rather than the other.

***Poisson regression.*** Poisson regression is mainly used to study waiting times or time between rare events.

## Watch out for...

Regression should not be used to make predictions outside of the range of the original data. In the example above, we can only make predictions from blood glucoses which are between 5 and 20.

## Regression or correlation?

Regression and correlation are easily confused.

Correlation measures the *strength* of the association between variables.

Regression *quantifies* the association. It is usually only used if one of the variables is thought to precede or cause the other.

## Ch 18 SURVIVAL ANALYSIS: LIFE TABLES AND KAPLAN–MEIER PLOTS

### How important are they?

Survival analysis techniques are used in just under 20% of papers.

### How easy are they to understand?

Life tables are difficult to interpret. Luckily, most papers make it easy for you by showing the resulting plots – these graphs give a good visual feel of what has happened to a population over time.

### When are they used?

Survival analysis techniques are concerned with representing the time until a single event occurs. That event is often death, but it could be any other single event, for example time until discharge from hospital.

Survival analysis techniques are able to deal with situations in which the end event has not happened in every patient or when information on a case is only known for a limited duration – known as "censored" observations.

### What do they mean?

*Life table.* A life table is a table of the proportion of patients surviving over time.

Life table methods look at the data at a number of fixed time points and calculate the survival rate at those times. The most commonly used method is Kaplan–Meier.

### Kaplan–Meier

The Kaplan–Meier approach recalculates the survival rate when an end event (e.g. death) occurs in the data set, i.e. when a change happens rather than at fixed intervals.

This is usually represented as a "survival plot". *Fig. 13* shows a fictitious example.

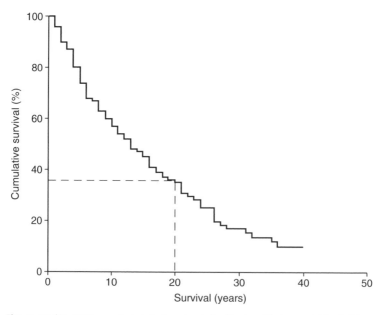

**Fig. 13.** Kaplan–Meier survival plot of a cohort of patients with rheumatoid arthritis.

The dashed line shows that at 20 years, 36% of this group of patients were still alive.

## Watch out for...

Life tables and Kaplan–Meier survival estimates are also used to compare survival between groups. The plots make any difference between survival in two groups beautifully clear. *Fig. 14* shows the same group of patients as above, but compares survival for men and women.

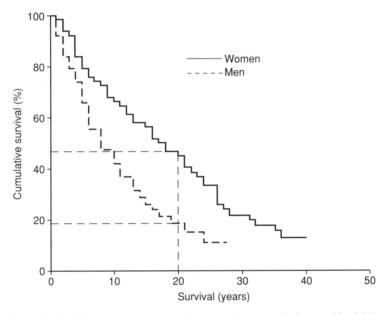

**Fig. 14.** Kaplan–Meier survival plot comparing men and women with rheumatoid arthritis.

In this example 46% of women were still alive at 20 years but only 18% of men.

Each time an observation is censored, the remaining cohort gets smaller. The reliability of the survival estimates therefore reduce with time.

The test to compare the survival between these two groups is called the "log rank test". Its *P* value will tell you how significant the result of the test is.

# Ch 19 THE COX REGRESSION MODEL

Also known as the "Cox proportional hazards survival model".

## How important is it?

It appeared in one in five papers.

## How easy is it to understand?

 Just aim to understand the end result – the "hazard ratio" (HR).

## When is it used?

The Cox regression model is used to investigate the relationship between an event (usually death) and possible explanatory variables, for instance smoking status or weight.

## What does it mean?

The Cox regression model provides us with estimates of the effect that different factors have on the time until the end event.

As well as considering the significance of the effect of different factors (e.g. how much shorter male life expectancy is compared to that of women), the model can give us an estimate of life expectancy for an individual (for example, a 60 year old woman with ischaemic heart disease, or a 40 year old man who smokes).

The HR is the ratio of the chance (the "hazard") of an event in one group of observations divided by the chance (hazard) of the event in another group. A hazard ratio of 1 means the risk is 1 × that of the second group, i.e. the same. An HR of 2 implies twice the risk.

**EXAMPLE**

The Cox regression model shows us the effect of being in one group compared with another.

Using the rheumatoid arthritis cohort in *Fig. 13*, we can calculate the effect that gender has on survival. *Table 6* gives the results of a Cox regression model estimate of the effect.

**Table 6.** Cox regression model estimate of the effect of sex on survival in a cohort of patients with rheumatoid arthritis

| Parameter | HR[a] (95% CI)[b] | df [c] | P value[d] |
|---|---|---|---|
| Sex (Male) | 1.91 (1.21 to 3.01) | 1 | <0.05 |

[a] The HR of 1.91 means that the risk of death in any particular time period for men was 1.91 times that for women.

[b] This CI means we can be 95% confident that the true HR is between 1.21 and 3.01.

[c] Degrees of freedom – see *Glossary*.

[d] The *P* value of <0.05 suggests that the result is significant.

# Ch 20 SENSITIVITY, SPECIFICITY AND PREDICTIVE VALUE

### How important are they?

**⊗⊗**  While discussed in only 10% of papers, a working knowledge is important in interpreting papers that study screening.

### How easy are they to understand?

  The tables themselves are fairly easy to understand. However, there is a bewildering array of information that can be derived from them.

To avoid making your head spin, do not read this section until you are feeling fresh. You may need to go over it a few days running until it is clear in your mind.

### When are they used?

They are used to analyze the value of screening or tests.

### What do they mean?

Think of any screening test for a disease. For each patient:

- the disease itself may be present or absent;

- the test result may be positive or negative.

We need to know how useful the test is.

The results can be put in the "two-way table" shown in *Table 7*. Try working through it.

**Table 7.** Two-way table

|  |  | Disease: |  |
|---|---|---|---|
|  |  | Present | Absent |
| Test result: | Positive | A | B (False positive) |
|  | Negative | C (False negative) | D |

**Sensitivity.** If a patient has the disease, we need to know how often the test will be positive, i.e. "positive in disease".

This is calculated from: $\dfrac{A}{A + C}$

This is the rate of pick-up of the disease in a test, and is called the *Sensitivity*.

**Specificity.** If the patient is in fact healthy, we want to know how often the test will be negative, i.e. "negative in health".

This is given by: $\dfrac{D}{D + B}$

This is the rate at which a test can exclude the possibility of the disease , and is known as the *Specificity*.

**Positive Predictive Value.** If the test result is positive, what is the likelihood that the patient will have the condition?

Look at: $\dfrac{A}{A + B}$

This is known as the *Positive Predictive Value* (PPV).

***Negative Predictive Value.*** If the test result is negative, what is the likelihood that the patient will be healthy?

Here we use:  $\dfrac{D}{D + C}$

This is known as the *Negative Predictive Value* (NPV).

In a perfect test, the sensitivity, specificity, PPV and NPV would each have a value of 1. The lower the value (the nearer to zero), the less useful the test is in that respect.

## EXAMPLES

Confused? Try working through an example.

Imagine a blood test for gastric cancer, tried out on 100 patients admitted with haematemesis. The actual presence or absence of gastric cancers was diagnosed from endoscopic findings and biopsy. The results are shown in *Table 8*.

**Table 8.** Two-way table for blood test for gastric cancer

|               |          | Gastric cancer: | |
| --- | --- | --- | --- |
|               |          | Present | Absent |
| Blood result: | Positive | 20 | 30 |
|               | Negative | 5  | 45 |

Sensitivity $= \dfrac{20}{20 + 5} = \dfrac{20}{25} = 0.8$

If the gastric cancer is present, there is an 80% (0.8) chance of the test picking it up.

Specificity $= \dfrac{45}{30 + 45} = \dfrac{45}{75} = 0.6$

If there is no gastric cancer there is a 60% (0.6) chance of the test being negative – but 40% will have a false positive result.

$$PPV = \frac{20}{20 + 30} = \frac{20}{50} = 0.4$$

There is a 40% (0.4) chance, if the test is positive, that the patient actually has gastric cancer.

$$NPV = \frac{45}{45 + 5} = \frac{45}{50} = 0.9$$

There is a 90% (0.9) chance, if the test is negative, that the patient does not have gastric cancer. However, there is still a 10% chance of a false negative, i.e. that the patient does have gastric cancer.

## Likelihood ratios

One more set of ratios to know about.

Before any testing, there is a background probability of a patient having a condition, known as the "pre-test probability". The test helps us to move our suspicion one way or the other, giving us a "post-test probability". The "likelihood ratio" (LR) gives a value to how much that probability changes once we know the test result.

"LR+" is the multiplier for how much more likely a patient is to have the condition if the test result is positive. To calculate LR+, divide the sensitivity by (1 – specificity).

Head spinning again? Try using the example above to calculate the LR for a positive result:

$$LR+ = \frac{\text{probability that a patient } \textit{with} \text{ the disease has a } \textit{positive} \text{ result}}{\text{probability that a patient } \textit{without} \text{ the disease has a } \textit{positive} \text{ result}}$$

$$= \frac{\text{sensitivity}}{(1 - \text{sensitivity})} = \frac{0.8}{1 - 0.6} = \frac{0.8}{0.4} = 2$$

So, if the test result is positive, the chances that the patient actually has gastric cancer have doubled.

"LR–" is the multiplier for how much the risk of having the condition has *decreased* if the test is *negative*. For the same test:

$$LR- = \frac{\text{probability that a patient } \textit{with} \text{ the disease has a } \textit{negative} \text{ result}}{\text{probability that a patient } \textit{without} \text{ the disease has a } \textit{negative} \text{ result}}$$

$$= \frac{(1 - \text{sensitivity})}{\text{sensitivity}} = \frac{1 - 0.8}{0.6} = \frac{0.2}{0.6} = 0.33$$

Here, when the screening test result is negative, the risk for that patient of having gastric cancer is a third of his pre-test probability.

LRs can range from zero to infinity. The higher the LR is above 1, the higher the likelihood of disease. The closer the LR is to 0, the less likely the disease. Tests whose LRs are close to 1 lack diagnostic value.

## Watch out for...

Tip: Invent an imaginary screening or diagnostic test of your own, fill the boxes in and work out the various values. Then change the results to make the test a lot less or more effective and see how it affects the values.

One thing you may notice is that in a rare condition, even a diagnostic test with a very high sensitivity may have a low PPV.

If you are still feeling confused, you are in good company. Many colleagues far brighter than us admit that they get confused over sensitivity, PPV etc.

Try copying the following summary into your diary and refer to it when reading a paper:

- **Sensitivity:** how often the test is positive if the patient has the disease.

- **Specificity:** if the patient is healthy, how often the test will be negative.

- **PPV:** If the test is positive, the likelihood that the patient has the condition.

- **NPV:** If the test is negative, the likelihood that the patient will be healthy.

- **LR+:** The multiplier for the pre-test likelihood of a patient having the condition if the test is positive.

- **LR−:** The multiplier for the pre-test likelihood of a patient not having the condition if the test is negative.

Examiners love to give a set of figures which you can turn into a two-way table and ask you to calculate sensitivity, PPV etc. from them. Keep practising until you are comfortable at working with these values.

## Ch 21 LEVEL OF AGREEMENT

### How important is it?

✪ Not often used.

### How easy is it to understand?

### When is it used?

It is a comparison of how well people or tests agree.

Typically it is used to look at how accurately a test can be repeated.

### What does it mean?

The level of agreement can vary from zero to 1.

An agreement of zero means that there is no significant agreement – no more than would have been expected by chance.

An agreement of 0.5 or more is considered a good agreement; a value of 0.7 shows very good agreement.

An agreement of 1 means that there is perfect agreement.

For "continuous variables" (those that can take any value within a given range, for instance blood glucose readings), a commonly used measure of agreement is the "intra-class correlation coefficient" (ICC).

When data can be put in ordered categories ("ordinal data"), the "kappa" statistic (often written as κ) is often used.

**EXAMPLE**

The same cervical smear slides were examined by the cytology departments of two hospitals. Both laboratories put each slide into one of the following ordered categories: normal, CIN 1, CIN 2, CIN 3, and invasive cancer. Kappa was 0.3, suggesting that there was little agreement between the two laboratories.

## Watch out for...

Measures of agreement are different to correlation. If two clinicians, for example, independently perform mini mental state examinations, and one consistently gives scores that are five points above those of the other, the correlation will be high. However, the agreement score would be very low.

The level of agreement may be given with its *P* value (see *Chapter 9*). However, the significance gives no indication of the importance of the level of agreement.

# Ch 22 OTHER CONCEPTS

## Multiple testing adjustment

Importance:
Ease of understanding: 👍👍

One fundamental principle of statistics is that we accept there is a chance we will come to the wrong conclusion. If we reject a null hypothesis with a *P* value of 0.05, then there is still the 5% possibility that we should not have rejected the hypothesis and therefore a 5% chance that we have come to the wrong conclusion.

If we do lots of testing then this chance of making a mistake will be present each time we do a test and therefore the more tests we do the greater the chances of drawing the wrong conclusion.

Multiple testing adjustment techniques therefore adjust the *P* value to keep the overall chance of coming to the wrong conclusion at a certain level (usually 5%).

The most commonly used method is the "Bonferroni" adjustment.

## 1- and 2-tailed tests

Importance:
Ease of understanding: 👍

When trying to reject a "null hypothesis" (described further in *Chapter 9*), we are generally interested in two possibilities: either we can reject it because the new treatment is better than the current one, or because it is worse. By allowing the null hypothesis to be rejected from either direction we are performing a "two-tailed test" – we are rejecting it when the result is in either "tail" of the test distribution.

Occasionally there are situations where we are only interested in rejecting a hypothesis if the new treatment is worse that the current one but not if it is better. This would be better analyzed with a one-tailed test. However, be very sceptical of one-tailed tests. A $P$ value that is not quite significant on a two-tailed test may become significant if a one-tailed test is used. Authors have been known to use this to their advantage!

## Incidence

Importance: ✪✪✪
Ease of understanding: 👍👍👍👍

The number of **new** cases of a condition **over a given time** as a percentage of the population.

Example: Each year 15 people in a practice of 1000 patients develop Brett's palsy.

$$\frac{15}{1000} \times 100 = \text{yearly incidence of } 1.5\%$$

To compare the incidence rates of two groups over a period of time, the "incidence rate ratio" is used.

## Prevalence (= Point Prevalence Rate)

Importance ✪✪✪
Ease of understanding: 👍👍👍👍

The **existing** number of cases of a condition at **a single point in time** as a percentage of the population.

Example: At the time of a study 90 people in a practice of 1000 patients were suffering from Brett's palsy (15 diagnosed in the last year plus 75 diagnosed in previous years).

$$\frac{90}{1000} \times 100 = \text{a prevalence of } 9\%$$

With chronic diseases like the fictitious Brett's palsy, the incidence will be lower than the prevalence – each year's new diagnoses swell the number of existing cases.

With short-term illnesses the opposite may be true. 75% of a population may have a cold each year (incidence), but at any moment only 2% are actually suffering (prevalence).

Check that you can explain the difference between incidence and prevalence.

## Power

Importance: ✪✪
Ease of understanding: 👍👍👍

The power of a study is the probability that it would detect a statistically significant difference.

If the difference expected is 100% cure compared with 0% cure with previous treatments, a very small study would have sufficient power to detect that.

However if the expected difference is much smaller, e.g. 1%, then a much larger sample size would be needed to get sufficient power to produce a result with statistical significance.

## Bayesian statistics

Importance: ✪
Ease of understanding: 👍

Bayesian analysis is not often used. It is a totally different statistical approach to the classical, "frequentist" statistics explained in this book.

In Bayesian statistics, rather than considering the sample of data on its own, a "prior distribution" is set up using information that is already available. For instance, the researcher may give a numerical value and weighting to previous opinion and experience as well as previous research findings.

One consideration is that different researchers may put different weighting on the same previous findings.

The new sample data are then used to adjust this prior information to form a "posterior distribution". Thus these resulting figures have taken *both* the disparate old data *and* the new data into account.

Bayesian methodology is intuitively appealing because it reflects how we think. When we read about a new study we do not consider its results in isolation, we factor it in to our pre-existing opinions, knowledge and experience of dealing with patients.

It is only recently that computer power has been sufficient to calculate the complex models that are needed for Bayesian analysis.

## Ch 23 INTRODUCTION

In this section we have given five real-life examples of how researchers use statistical techniques to describe and analyze their work.

The extracts have been taken from research papers published in *The Lancet*, the *British Medical Journal*, *BJU International*, the *New England Journal of Medicine*, and the *Journal of the American Medical Association*. If you want to see the original papers, you can download them from, respectively:

- www.thelancet.com
- www.bmj.com
- www.bjuinternational.com
- www.nejm.org
- jama.jamanetwork.com/journal.aspx

We have made minor alterations to the abstracts to make them easier to follow, but the data have not been changed.

If you wish, you can use this part to test what you have learnt:

- First, go through the abstracts and results and note down what statistical techniques have been used.
- Then try to work out why the authors have used those techniques.
- Next, try to interpret the results.
- Finally, check out your understanding by comparing it with our commentary.

# Ch 24 MEDIANS, INTERQUARTILE RANGES AND ODDS RATIOS

The following extract is reproduced with permission from Elsevier.

Adapted from:

Fazel S, Wolf A, Långström N, Newton C, Lichtenstein P. Premature mortality in epilepsy and the role of psychiatric comorbidity: a total population study. *Lancet*, 2013;382:1646–54. doi:10.1016/S0140-6736(13)60899-5.

## Summary

**Background:** Epilepsy is associated with high rates of premature mortality, but the contribution of psychiatric comorbidity is uncertain. We assessed the prevalence and risks of premature mortality from external causes such as suicide, accidents, and assaults in people with epilepsy with and without psychiatric comorbidity.

**Methods:** We studied all individuals born in Sweden between 1954 and 2009 with inpatient and outpatient diagnoses of epilepsy (n=69 995) for risks and causes of premature mortality. Patients were compared with age-matched and sex-matched general population controls (n=660 869) and unaffected siblings (n=81 396).

**Findings:** 6155 (8.8%) people with epilepsy died during follow-up, at a median age of 34.5 (IQR 21.0–44.0) years with substantially elevated odds of premature mortality (adjusted odds ratio [aOR] of 11.1 [95% CI 10.6–11.6] compared with general population controls, and 11.4 [10.4–12.5] compared with unaffected siblings). Of those deaths, 15.8% (n=972) were from external causes. Of those who died from external causes, 75.2% (n=731) had comorbid psychiatric disorders.

## What statistical methods were used and why?

The authors wanted to explore the causes of the high *incidence* of premature mortality in people with epilepsy.

They therefore analyzed a large cohort of patients for risks and causes of premature mortality, and compared them with controls. They calculated the *percentage* of patients who died during follow-up. They also worked out the *median* age of death, with its *interquartile range* (IQR), and used *odds ratios* (OR) to compare the *odds* of premature death with that of the control groups. The data were "adjusted" for age, sex and socio-demographic confounders to allow direct comparison.

The authors wanted to give the ranges that were likely to contain the true odds ratios, so gave them with their 95% *confidence intervals* (CI).

## What do the results mean?

The average age of death of those that died during follow-up was given as a median. This means that half the patients were aged 34.5 or over when they died, and half were below that age. The use of the median (rather than the mean) suggests that the distribution of ages at death was *skewed*.

The IQR of 21.0–44.0 means that a quarter of those patients were aged under 21 (the 1st quartile point), a quarter were 44 or older (the 3rd quartile point), and the other half were aged between 21 and 44.

The summary states that 6155 out of 69 995 people with epilepsy died before the end of the follow-up period. This gives an incidence, or mortality rate, of:

$$\frac{6155}{69\,995} \times 100 = 8.8\%$$

This can be expressed in terms of the odds of premature death:

$$\frac{\text{number of deaths}}{\text{number surviving}} = \frac{6155}{(69\,995 - 6155)} = \frac{6155}{63\,840} = 0.0964$$

Out of 660 869 controls, 4892 died prematurely, an incidence of:

$$\frac{4892}{(660\,869)} \times 100 = 0.74\%$$

Converting this into the odds of premature death for the controls:

$$\frac{\text{number of deaths}}{\text{number surviving}} = \frac{4892}{(660\,869 - 4892)} = \frac{4892}{65\,5977} = 0.00746$$

The unadjusted odds ratio is therefore:

$$\frac{\text{odds of death in patients with epilepsy}}{\text{odds of death in controls}} = \frac{0.0964}{0.00746} = 12.9$$

After adjusting for age, sex and socio-demographic confounders, the authors calculated the odds ratio to be 11.1. This indicates that the risk of premature death in patients with epilepsy was eleven times that of the control population.

The 95% CI of 10.6–11.6 is the range in which the true value (i.e. the odds ratio if they had studied an infinite number of patients) is likely to be. As the CI for the odds ratio doesn't include 1 (no difference in odds), the difference between the odds of death in this study is statistically significant.

The adjusted OR between patients with epilepsy and their unaffected siblings was 11.4. Again, the OR of >1 indicates an increased risk for patients with epilepsy. The fact that the 95% CI for the OR is 10.4–12.5, and doesn't include 1, indicates that this result is also significant.

Of the 6155 deaths in patients with epilepsy, 972 were from external causes, giving a percentage of:

$$\frac{972}{6155} \times 100 = 15.8\%$$

Of those 972 who died from external causes, 731 had comorbid psychiatric disorders:

$$\frac{731}{972} \times 100 = 75.2\%$$

The authors concluded that their results indicate high rates of premature mortality in people with epilepsy, with psychiatric comorbidity making a substantial contribution to this mortality.

## Ch 25 RISK RATIOS AND NUMBER NEEDED TO TREAT

The following extract is reproduced with permission from The BMJ Publishing Group Ltd.

Adapted from:

Marschall J, Carpenter C, Fowler S, Trautner B. Antibiotic prophylaxis for urinary tract infections after removal of urinary catheter: meta-analysis. *BMJ*, 2013;346:f3147. doi: 10.1136/bmj.f3147

### Abstract

**Objective:** To determine whether antibiotic prophylaxis at the time of removal of a urinary catheter reduces the risk of subsequent symptomatic urinary tract infection.

**Design:** Systematic review and meta-analysis of studies published before November 2012 identified through PubMed, Embase, Scopus, and the Cochrane Library.

**Inclusion criteria:** Studies were included if they examined antibiotic prophylaxis administered to prevent symptomatic urinary tract infection after removal of a short term ($\leq$14 days) urinary catheter.

**Results:** Seven controlled studies had symptomatic urinary tract infection after catheter removal as an endpoint; six were randomized controlled trials and one was a non-randomized controlled intervention study. The incidence of symptomatic urinary tract infection was 4.7%

(31/665) in the antibiotic prophylaxis group v 10.5% (90/855) in the control group.

Overall, antibiotic prophylaxis was associated with benefit to the patient, with an absolute reduction in risk of urinary tract infection of 5.8% between intervention and control groups. The risk ratio was 0.45 (95% confidence interval 0.28 to 0.72). The number needed to treat to prevent one urinary tract infection was 17 (12 to 30).

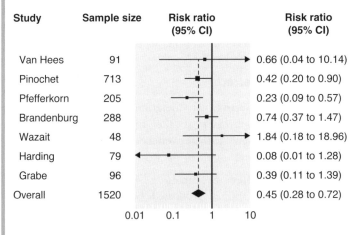

| Study | Sample size | Risk ratio (95% CI) | Risk ratio (95% CI) |
|---|---|---|---|
| Van Hees | 91 | | 0.66 (0.04 to 10.14) |
| Pinochet | 713 | | 0.42 (0.20 to 0.90) |
| Pfefferkorn | 205 | | 0.23 (0.09 to 0.57) |
| Brandenburg | 288 | | 0.74 (0.37 to 1.47) |
| Wazait | 48 | | 1.84 (0.18 to 18.96) |
| Harding | 79 | | 0.08 (0.01 to 1.28) |
| Grabe | 96 | | 0.39 (0.11 to 1.39) |
| Overall | 1520 | | 0.45 (0.28 to 0.72) |

**Fig. 15.** Forest plot of seven included studies with 1520 participants on effect of antibiotic prophylaxis on urinary tract infections after removal of urinary catheter.

## What statistical methods were used and why?

The authors performed a *meta-analysis* of controlled trials, combining the results of the individual trials to find out whether antibiotic prophylaxis at the time of urinary catheter removal prevents some subsequent symptomatic urinary tract infections (UTIs).

The *risk ratios* and *confidence intervals* for each of the seven studies were shown in a *Forest plot*, with a diamond and dotted line indicating the *combined estimate*.

The researchers calculated the *incidence* of UTIs in the two groups, giving that *risk* as a *percentage*. They used a *risk ratio* to compare those risks. They also gave the *absolute risk reduction*, as well as the *number needed to treat* to prevent one UTI.

The researchers wanted to give the range that was likely to contain the true risk ratio and number needed to treat, so gave them with their 95% *confidence intervals*.

## What do the results mean?

In the antibiotic prophylaxis group, 31 out of 665 patients developed a UTI. As a percentage:

$$\text{Incidence} = \frac{31}{665} \times 100 = 4.7\%$$

This is the same as the risk, or probability, that a UTI would happen in this group.

In the control group, 90 out of 855 subsequently had a UTI:

$$\text{Incidence (risk)} = \frac{90}{855} \times 100 = 10.5\%$$

The risk ratio was calculated by dividing the risk in the antibiotic group with that in the control group:

$$\frac{4.7}{10.5} = 0.45$$

This risk ratio of <1 shows that the risk of UTIs in the antibiotic prophylaxis group was lower than that in the control group.

The 95% confidence interval (CI) of 0.28 to 0.72 does not include 1 (no difference in risk), so it is statistically significant.

The Forest plot shows the diversity of the risk ratios from different studies, including one study (Wazait) that showed a higher UTI risk in the antibiotic group. The risk ratios of five of the studies had 95% CIs that included 1, so were in themselves not statistically significant. The combined risk ratio and 95% CI (calculated above) are given on the line labelled "Overall".

From the study results, we can confirm the authors' calculations for the absolute risk reduction (ARR) and the number needed to treat (NNT). We can also calculate the relative risk reduction (RRR).

ARR = [risk in the control group] − [risk in the antibiotic group] = 10.5% − 4.7% = 5.8%

The NNT is the number of patients who need to be treated for one to get benefit:

$$\text{NNT} = \frac{100}{\text{ARR}} = \frac{100}{5.8} = 17$$

The range in which we can be 95% confident that the "true value" for the NNT lies has been calculated to be 12 to 30.

The RRR is the percentage by which the intervention reduces the event rate:

$$\frac{10.5-4.7}{10.5} = \frac{5.8}{10.5} = 0.55 = 55\%$$

The researchers concluded that adults given antibiotic prophylaxis at the time of urinary catheter removal were significantly less likely to have a UTI than controls, with an NNT to prevent infection of 17.

# Ch 26 CORRELATION AND REGRESSION

The following extract is reproduced with permission from John Wiley and Sons.

Adapted from:

Loke T, Sevfi D, Khadra M. Prostate cancer incidence in Australia correlates inversely with solar radiation. *BJU International*, 2011;108(s2):66–70. doi: 10.1111/j.1464-410X.2011.10736.x.

## Abstract

**Objective:** To ascertain if prostate cancer incidence rates correlate with solar radiation among non-urban populations of men in Australia.

**Patients and methods:** Local government areas from each state and territory were selected using explicit criteria. Urban areas were excluded from analysis.

For each local government area, prostate cancer incidence rates and averaged long-term solar radiation were obtained.

The strength of the association between prostate cancer incidence and solar radiation was determined.

**Results:** Among 70 local government areas of Australia, age-standardized prostate cancer incidence rates for the period 1998–2007 correlated inversely with daily solar radiation averaged over the last two decades.

**Conclusion:** There exists an association between less solar radiation and higher prostate cancer incidence in Australia.

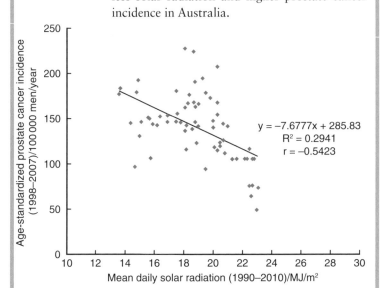

Fig. 16. Age-standardized prostate cancer incidence vs. mean daily solar radiation.

A line of best fit was derived using least-squares regression. $R^2$ was 0.294 (95% CI 0.120, 0.468) and the Pearson correlation coefficient ($r$) was –0.542, with a two-tailed $P < 0.001$.

## What statistical methods were used and why?

The researchers wanted to know whether there was a relationship between prostate cancer incidence and sun exposure, so needed to measure the *correlation* between the two.

They found that the data had a *normal distribution*, so used the *Pearson correlation coefficient* as a measure of the correlation.

It may be that the association could be causal, i.e. that sun exposure is protective against prostate cancer, so the authors calculated the *line of best fit* through the scatter of points (the *regression line*), as well as the *regression equation* with its *regression coefficient* and *regression constant*.

## What do the results mean?

The Pearson correlation coefficient for sun exposure and prostate cancer incidence is given as $r = -0.542$. This $r$ value indicates a reasonable *negative* correlation.

$P < 0.001$ indicates that an $r$ value of $-0.542$ (or even more negative) would have happened by chance less than 1 in 1000 times if there were really no correlation.

*Figure 16* shows the authors' *regression graph* comparing mean solar radiation with prostate cancer incidence. Each dot represents the values for one area of Australia. The line through the dots is the *regression line*.

The authors show the *regression equation* in the graph: $y = -7.6777x + 285.83$

In this equation:

x (the horizontal axis of the graph) indicates the *mean* solar daily radiation.

y (the vertical axis of the graph) indicates the *incidence* of prostate cancer per 100 000 men per year.

The *regression constant* of 285.83 is the point at which the regression line would hit the vertical axis of the graph (when mean solar daily radiation = 0).

The *regression coefficient* gives the gradient of the line: the incidence of prostate cancer reduces by 7.6777 for every unit increase ($MJ/m^2$) in mean daily solar radiation.

The authors therefore suggested that their analysis adds to evidence in support of a protective effect of solar radiation in prostate cancer.

# Ch 27 SURVIVAL ANALYSIS

Adapted from:

Imazio M, Brucato A, Cemin R, Ferrua S, *et al.* A randomized trial of colchicine for acute pericarditis. *N Engl J Med.* 2013; 369:1522–8. DOI: 10.1056/NEJMoa1208536

## Abstract

**Background:** Colchicine is effective for the treatment of recurrent pericarditis. However, conclusive data are lacking regarding the use of colchicine during a first attack of acute pericarditis and in the prevention of recurrent symptoms.

**Methods:** In a multicenter, double-blind trial, eligible adults with acute pericarditis were randomly assigned to receive either colchicine or placebo in addition to conventional anti-inflammatory therapy with aspirin or ibuprofen. The primary study outcome was incessant or recurrent pericarditis.

**Results:** A total of 240 patients were enrolled, and 120 were randomly assigned to each of the two study groups. The primary outcome occurred in 20 patients (16.67%) in the colchicine group and 45 patients (37.5%) in the placebo group (relative risk reduction in the colchicine group, 0.56; 95% confidence interval, 0.30 to 0.72; number needed to treat, 4; $P<0.001$).

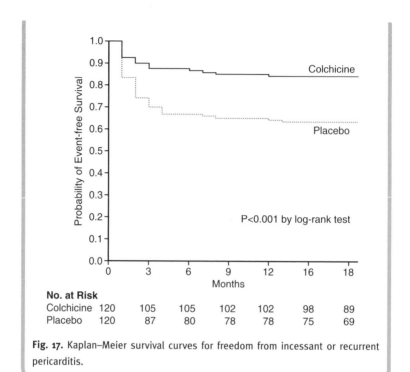

**Fig. 17.** Kaplan–Meier survival curves for freedom from incessant or recurrent pericarditis.

## What statistical methods were used and why?

The authors wanted to find out whether colchicine reduces the rate of recurrent pericarditis when used in a first episode of acute pericarditis.

The *null hypothesis* was that there was no difference between the group receiving colchicine and those not receiving it.

The *Kaplan-Meier survival curve* (*Fig. 17*) was used to give a visual representation of the probability of freedom from recurrent pericarditis over time in each group. The risk of recurrent pericarditis after 18 months of follow-up was compared using the *relative risk reduction*.

Pericarditis-free survival between the two groups was compared using the *log rank test*, with its 95% *confidence interval*. The likelihood that there was no real difference between the groups was given by the *P value*.

The number of patients who needed to be treated for one to get benefit was given by the *number needed to treat*.

## What do the results mean?

The risk of recurrent pericarditis in the colchicine group was 20/120, which is 16.67%. The risk in the other group was 45/120, which is 37.5%.

Colchicine therefore reduced the risk from 37.5% to 16.67%.

Absolute risk reduction (ARR) = 37.5 – 16.67 = 20.83%

Relative risk reduction $= \dfrac{ARR}{37.5} = \dfrac{20.83}{37.5} = 0.56$, which is 56%

Number needed to treat $= \dfrac{100}{ARR} = \dfrac{100}{20.83} = 4.8$

In the abstract, the authors have given this NNT as 4.

$P < 0.001$, so the probability of the difference having happened by chance is less than 0.001 in 1, i.e. less than 1 in 1000.

As $P < 0.05$, this is considered to be statistically significant.

This is stated another way by giving the 95% confidence interval. The CI of 0.30 to 0.72 does not include 1 (no difference in risk), again demonstrating statistical significance.

The conclusion was that colchicine reduced the rate of recurrent pericarditis.

# Ch 28 SENSITIVITY, SPECIFICITY AND PREDICTIVE VALUES

Adapted from:

Perry J, Stiell I, Sivilotti M, Bullard M, *et al*. Clinical decision rules to rule out subarachnoid hemorrhage for acute headache. *JAMA*, 2013;310: 1248–55. doi:10.1001/jama.2013.278018

## Abstract

**Importance:** Three clinical decision rules were previously derived to identify patients with headache requiring investigations to rule out subarachnoid haemorrhage (SAH).

**Objective:** To assess the accuracy, reliability, acceptability, and potential refinement (i.e. to improve sensitivity or specificity) of these rules in a new cohort of patients with headache.

**Design, setting, and patients:** Multicentre cohort study conducted at 10 university-affiliated Canadian tertiary care emergency departments from April 2006 to July 2010. Enrolled patients were 2131 adults with a headache peaking within 1 hour and no neurologic deficits.

**Main outcomes and measures:** Subarachnoid haemorrhage, defined as (1) subarachnoid blood on computed tomography scan; (2) xanthochromia in cerebrospinal fluid; or (3) red blood cells in the final tube of cerebrospinal fluid, with positive angiography findings.

**Results:** Of the 2131 enrolled patients, 132 had subarachnoid haemorrhage. Adding "thunderclap headache" (i.e. instantly peaking pain) and "limited neck flexion on examination" to the decision rule including any of: age 40 years or older, neck pain or stiffness, witnessed loss of consciousness, or onset during exertion resulted in the Ottawa SAH Rule, with 100% (95% CI, 97.2–100.0%) sensitivity and 15.3% (95% CI, 13.8–16.9%) specificity.

**Table 9.** Two-way table of number of patients categorised as having subarachnoid haemorrhage by clinical decision tool and by gold standard tests (given in "Main outcomes and measures" paragraph above)

|  |  | Outcome of gold standard tests | | Total |
|---|---|---|---|---|
|  |  | Positive | Negative |  |
| **Result from Ottawa SAH Rule** | **Positive** | 132 | 1694 | 1826 |
|  | **Negative** | 0 | 305 | 305 |
| **Total** |  | 132 | 1999 | 2131 |

Table derived from data given in the paper.

## What statistical methods were used and why?

The researchers wanted to know whether they could improve their existing clinical decision rules for ruling out subarachnoid haemorrhage. They decided whether patients had actually had a subarachnoid haemorrhage by using the "gold standard" tests that they listed in the abstract.

*Sensitivity* and *specificity* were used to give the value of their clinical decision rules, with their *95% confidence intervals*. They express these values as *percentages*.

We have simplified the abstract by removing the results of the pre-existing rules, and have used a *two-way table* to show the results (*Table 9*).

## What do the results mean?

In a perfect test, the sensitivity, specificity and predictive values would each have a value of 1. The lower the value (the nearer to zero), the less useful the decision rule is in that respect.

Sensitivity shows the rate of pick-up of the disease – if a patient has had a subarachnoid haemorrhage, it shows how often the Ottawa SAH Rule will be positive. This is calculated from:

$$\text{Sensitivity} = \frac{132}{132} = 1, \text{ or } 100\%.$$

So, if a patient has had a subarachnoid haemorrhage, the decision rule will always be positive.

The 95% confidence interval of 97.2–100% is the range in which the true value (i.e. the sensitivity if we treated an infinite number of patients) is likely to be.

Specificity is the rate at which the rule can exclude a subarachnoid haemorrhage – if the patient has not had one, it shows how often the decision rule will be negative. This is given by:

$$\text{Specificity} = \frac{305}{1999} = 0.153, \text{ or } 15.3\%.$$

This means that the decision will only be negative in 15 out of every 100 patients who have *not* had a subarachnoid haemorrhage.

The range in which the true value of the specificity is likely to be is given by the 95% confidence interval: 97.2–100%.

In the paper, the authors also give the *negative predictive value*. This is the likelihood that a patient has had a subarachnoid haemorrhage if the decision rule is negative.

$$NPV = \frac{305}{305} = 1, \text{ or } 100\%$$

The NPV of 100% means that no patients who had a negative decision rule result were found to have had a subarachnoid haemorrhage, so potentially a negative rule result could be used to rule out SAH and avoid unnecessary further investigations.

We can also calculate the *positive predictive value*, which is the likelihood that a patient has had a subarachnoid haemorrhage if the decision rule is positive.

$$PPV = \frac{132}{1826} = 0.072, \text{ or } 7.2\%$$

So, in patients for whom the decision rule is positive, the incidence of subarachnoid haemorrhage is 7.2%. However, 93 in 100 patients with a positive rule result will not actually have had a subarachnoid haemorrhage.

It is also possible to use the sensitivity and specificity values to calculate the *likelihood ratios*.

LR+ is the multiplier for how much more likely a patient is to have had a subarachnoid haemorrhage if the Ottawa SAH Rule is positive.

$$LR+ = \frac{\text{sensitivity}}{(1 - \text{specificity})} = \frac{1}{1 - 0.153} = \frac{1}{0.847} = 1.18$$

So, if the decision rule result is positive in a patient, that patient is only 1.18 times more likely to have had a subarachnoid haemorrhage than if the result is negative.

LR– is the multiplier for how much the risk of the patient having had a subarachnoid haemorrhage has *decreased* if the decision rule is *negative*. Using our calculated values for sensitivity and specificity gives:

$$LR- = \frac{(1 - \text{sensitivity})}{\text{specificity}} = \frac{1 - 1}{0.153} = \frac{0}{0.153} = 0$$

This suggests that if the decision rule result for a patient is negative, the risk that they have had a subarachnoid haemorrhage is zero, however high their pre-test probability.

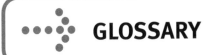

# GLOSSARY

Cross-references to other parts of the glossary are given in *italics*.

## Absolute risk reduction, ARR

The difference between the event *rate* in the intervention group and that in the control group. It is also the reciprocal of the *NNT*.

## Alpha, α

The alpha value is equivalent to the *P value* and should be interpreted in the same way.

## ANCOVA (ANalysis of COVAriance)

Analysis of covariance is an extension of *analysis of variance* (ANOVA) to allow for the inclusion of *continuous variables* in the model.

## ANOVA (ANalysis Of VAriance)

This is a group of statistical techniques used to compare the *means* of two of more samples to see whether they come from the same population. See *Chapter 10*.

## As prescribed analysis

In a controlled trial, this analysis evaluates participants by the treatment they actually receive, rather than what they were randomized to receive.

### Association

A word used to describe a relationship between two *variables*.

### Bar chart

In these graphs, the height of the bars represent the number of occurrences in each category. See *Chapter 6*.

### Beta, β

The beta value is the probability of accepting a *hypothesis* that is actually false. 1 – β is known as the *power* of the study.

### Bayesian statistics

An alternative way of analyzing data, it creates and combines numerical values for prior belief, existing data and new data. See *Chapter 22*.

### Binary variable

See *categorical variable* below.

### Bi-modal distribution

Where there are 2 *modes* in a set of data, the results are said to be bi-modal. See *Chapter 6*.

### Binomial distribution

When data can only take one of two values (for instance male or female), they are said to follow a binomial *distribution*.

## Bonferroni

A method that allows for the problems associated with making multiple comparisons. See *Chapter 22*.

## Box and whisker plot

A graph showing the *median*, *range* and *inter-quartile range* of a set of values. See *Chapter 5*.

## Case–control study

A retrospective study which investigates the relationship between an outcome and one or more risk factors. This is done by selecting patients who already have the disease or outcome *(cases)*, matching them to patients who do not (controls) and then comparing the effect of the risk factor(s) on the two groups. Compare this with *Cohort study*. See *Chapter 14*.

## Cases

This usually refers to patients but could refer to hospitals, wards, counties, blood samples etc.

## Categorical variable

A *variable* whose values represent different categories of the same feature. Examples include different blood groups, different eye colours, and different ethnic groups.

When the variable has only two categories, it is termed *"binary"* (e.g. gender). Where there is some inherent ordering (e.g. mild, moderate, severe), this is called an *"ordinal"* variable.

## Causation

The direct relationship of the cause to the effect that it produces, usually established in experimental studies.

## Censored

A censored observation is one where we do not have information for all of the observation period. This is usually seen in *survival analysis* where patients are followed for some time and then move away or withdraw consent for inclusion in the study. We cannot include them in the analysis after this point as we do not know what has happened to them. See *Chapter 18*.

## Central tendency

The "central" scores in a set of figures. *Mean*, *median* and *mode* are measures of central tendency.

## Chi-squared test, $\chi^2$

The chi-squared test is a test of association between two *categorical variables*. See *Chapter 12*.

## Cohort study

A prospective, observational study that follows a group (cohort) over a period of time and investigates the effect of a treatment or risk factor. Compare this with *case–control study*. See *Chapter 13*.

## Confidence interval, CI

A range of values within which we are fairly confident the true *population* value lies. For example, a 95% CI means that we can be 95% confident that the population value lies within those limits. See *Chapter 8*.

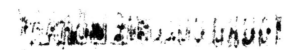

## Confounding

A confounding factor is the effect of a *covariate* or factor that cannot be separated out. For example, if women with a certain condition received a new treatment and men received placebo, it would not be possible to separate the treatment effect from the effect due to gender. Therefore gender would be a confounding factor.

## Continuous variable

A *variable* which can take any value within a given range, for instance BP. Compare this with *discrete variable*.

## Control charts

These are graphs used in *statistical process control*. They can give a visual early warning of when a measurement (for instance a ward infection rate) is changing and going outside a certain range.

## Correlation

When there is a linear relationship between two *variables* there is said to be a correlation between them. Examples are height and weight in children, or socio-economic class and mortality.

Measured on a scale from −1 (perfect negative correlation), through 0 (no relationship between the variables at all), to +1 (perfect positive correlation). See *Chapter 16*.

## Correlation coefficient

A measure of the strength of the linear relationship between two *variables*. See *Chapter 16*.

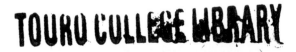

## Covariance

As with *correlation*, this describes the strength of a linear relationship between two variables. However, whereas correlation is measured on a scale from −1 to +1, so allowing direct comparison of different sets of data, covariance values can fall outside that range and cannot always be directly compared.

## Covariate

A covariate is a *continuous variable* that is not of primary interest but is measured because it may affect the outcome and may therefore need to be included in the analysis.

## Cox regression model

A method which explores the effects of different *variables* on survival. See *Chapter 19*.

## Database

A collection of records that is organized for ease and speed of retrieval.

## Degrees of freedom, df

The number of degrees of freedom, often abbreviated to df, is the number of independent pieces of information available for the statistician to make the calculations.

## Descriptive statistics

Descriptive statistics are those which describe the *data* in a *sample*. They include *means*, *medians*, *standard deviations*, *quartiles* and *histograms*. They are designed to give the reader an understanding of the data. Compare this with *inferential statistics*.

## Discrete variable

A *variable* where the data can only be certain values, usually whole numbers, for example the number of children in families. Compare this with *continuous variable*.

## Distribution

A distinct pattern of data may be considered as following a distribution. Many patterns of data have been described, the most useful of which is the *normal* distribution. See *Chapter 4*.

## Fisher's exact test

Fisher's exact test is an accurate test for association between *categorical variables*. See *Chapter 12*.

## Fields

See *variables* below.

## Hazard ratio, HR

The HR is the ratio of the hazard (chance of something harmful happening) of an event in one group of observations divided by the hazard of an event in a different group. An HR of 1 implies no difference in risk between the two groups, an HR of 2 implies double the risk. The HR should be stated with its *confidence intervals*. See *Chapter 19*.

## Histogram

A graph of *continuous* data with the data categorized into a number of classes. See example on *Chapter 6*.

## Hypothesis

A statement which can be tested that predicts the relationship between *variables*.

## Incidence

The rate or proportion of a group developing a condition within a given period.

## Inferential statistics

All statistical methods which test something are inferential. They estimate whether the results suggest that there is a real difference in the *populations*. Compare this with *descriptive statistics*.

## Intention to treat (ITT) analysis

In a controlled trial, this approach analyses participants according to the treatment arm they were randomized into, regardless of whether or not they actually received that intervention.

## Interaction

An interaction is when two or more *variables* are related to one another and therefore not acting independently.

## Inter-quartile range, IQR

A measure of spread given by the difference between the first *quartile* (the value below which 25% of the cases lie) and the third quartile (the value below which 75% of the cases lie). The IQR contains the middle half of the sample. See *Chapter 5*.

## Intra-class correlation coefficient

This correlation measures the *level of agreement* between two *continuous variables*. It is commonly used to look at how accurately a test can be repeated, for instance by different people. See *Chapter 21.*

## Kaplan–Meier survival plot

Kaplan–Meier plots are a method of graphically displaying the survival of a sample *cohort* of which the survival estimates are re-calculated whenever there is a death. See *Chapter 18.*

## Kappa, κ

This is a measure of the *level of agreement* between two *categorical* measures. It is often used to look at how accurately a test can be repeated, for instance by different people. See *Chapter 21.*

## Kolmogorov Smirnov test

Kolmogorov Smirnov tests the hypothesis that the collected data are from a *normal distribution*. It is therefore used to assess whether *parametric* statistics can be used. See *Chapter 10.*

## Kruskal Wallis test

This is a *non-parametric* test which compares two or more independent groups. See *Chapter 11.*

## Level of agreement

A comparison of how well people or tests agree. See *Chapter 21.*

## Life table

A table of the proportion of patients surviving over time. It is used in survival analysis. See *Chapter 18*.

## Likelihood ratio, LR

This is the likelihood that a test result would be expected in patients with a condition, divided by the likelihood that that same result would be expected in patients without that condition. See *Chapter 20*.

## Log rank test

A *non-parametric* test used for the comparison of survival estimates using *Kaplan–Meier* or *life table* estimates. See *Chapter 18*.

## Logistic regression

Logistic regression is a variation of *linear regression* that is used when there are only two possible outcomes. See *Chapter 17*.

## Mann–Whitney U test

A *non-parametric* test to see whether there is a significant difference between two sets of data that have come from two different sets of *subjects*. See *Chapter 11*.

## Mantel Haenszel test

An extension of the *chi-squared* test to compare several two-way tables. This technique can be applied in *meta-analysis*. See *Chapter 12*.

## Mean

The sum of the observed values divided by the number of observations. Compare this with *median* and *mode*. See *Chapter 4*.

## Median

The middle observation when the observed values are ranked from smallest to largest. Compare this with *mean* and *mode*. See *Chapter 5*.

## Meta-analysis

Meta-analysis is a method of combining results from a number of independent studies to give one overall estimate of effect. See *Chapter 8* for an example.

## Mode

The most commonly occurring observed value. Compare this with *mean* and *median*. See *Chapter 6*.

## Negative predictive value (NPV)

If a diagnostic test is negative, the NPV is the chance that a patient does not have the condition. Compare this with *positive predictive value*. See *Chapter 20*.

## Nominal data

Data that can be placed in named categories that have no particular order, for example eye colour.

## Non-parametric test

A test which is not dependent on the *distribution* (shape) of the data. See *Chapter 11*.

## Normal distribution

This refers to a *distribution* of data that is symmetrical. In a graph it forms a characteristic bell shape. See *Chapter 4*.

## Null hypothesis

A hypothesis that there is no difference between the groups being tested. The result of the test either supports or rejects that hypothesis.

Paradoxically, the null hypothesis is usually the opposite of what we are actually interested in finding out. If we want to know whether there is a difference between two treatments, then the null hypothesis would be that there is no difference. The statistical test is used to see whether this has been disproved. See *Chapter 9*.

## Number needed to harm, NNH

NNH is the number of patients that need to be treated for one to be harmed by the treatment. See *Chapter 15*.

## Number needed to treat, NNT

NNT is the number of patients that need to be treated for one to get benefit. See *Chapter 15*.

## Odds

The ratio of the number of times an event happens to the number of time it does not happen in a group of patients. Odds and *risk* give similar values when considering rare events (e.g. winning the lottery), but may be substantially different for common events (e.g. not winning the lottery!). See *Chapter 14*.

## Odds ratio (OR)

The *odds* of an event happening in one group, divided by the odds of it happening in another group. See *Chapter 14*.

## One-tailed test

A test where the *null hypothesis* can only be rejected in one direction, for example if new treatment is worse than current treatment but not if it is better. It should only rarely be used. Compare this with a *two-tailed test*. See *Chapter 22*.

## Ordinal data

Data that can be allocated to categories that can be "ordered", e.g. from least to strongest. An example is the staging of malignancy.

## *P* value

Usually used to test a *null hypothesis*, the *P* value gives the probability of any observed differences having happened by chance. See *Chapter 9*.

## Parametric test

Any test that has an assumption that the data need to to follow a certain distribution can be considered to be a parametric test. The most common distribution that the data need to follow is the *normal distribution*. Examples are the *t test* and ANOVA. See *Chapter 10*.

## Pearson correlation coefficient

A method of calculating a correlation coefficient if the values are sampled from a *normal* population. See *Chapter 16*.

## Percentage

The number of items in a category, divided by the total number in the group, then multiplied by 100. See *Chapter 3*.

## Per protocol (PP) analysis

In a controlled trial, this type of analysis only includes those participants who complete all stages of the study as defined in the protocol. It excludes participants who stopped taking their treatment.

## Poisson distribution

This *distribution* represents the number of events happening in a fixed time interval, for instance the number of deaths in a year.

## Poisson regression

A variation of *regression* calculations which allows for the frequency of rare events. See *Chapter 17*.

## Population

The complete set of subjects from which a sample is drawn.

## Positive predictive value, PPV

If a diagnostic test is positive, the PPV is the chance that a patient has the condition. Compare this with *negative predictive value*. See *Chapter 20*.

## Power

The power of a study is the probability that it will detect a statistically *significant* difference. See *Chapter 22*.

## Prevalence

The proportion of a group with a condition at a single point in time. See *Chapter 22*.

## Proportional hazards survival model

This is a group of survival analysis models. They assume that the risk of an event in one group is proportionately larger or smaller than the risk in the other group, and that this proportion does not change over time. The most commonly used example is the *Cox regression model*.

## Quartiles

A *median* value may be given with its quartiles. The $1^{st}$ quartile point has ¼ of the data below it, the $3^{rd}$ quartile has ¾ of the data below it. See *Chapter 5*.

## r

Where there is a linear relationship between two variables there is said to be a *correlation* between them. The *correlation coefficient* gives the strength of that relationship. See *Chapter 16*.

## R²

An estimate of the amount of the variation in the data that is being explained by a *correlation* or *regression* model. See Chapters 16 and 17.

## Range

The difference between the maximum and minimum score in a set of figures.

## Rank

A numerical value given to an observation showing its relative order in a set of data.

## Rate

The number of times that an event happens in a fixed period of time.

## Regression

Regression analysis is a technique for finding the relationship between two *variables*, one of which is dependent on the other. See *Chapter 17*.

## Relative risk

*Risk ratio* is often referred to as *relative risk*. However, *odds ratios* are also a measure of relative risk.

## Relative risk reduction, RRR

The proportion by which an intervention reduces the *risk* of an event. Compare this with *absolute risk reduction*. See *Chapter 15*.

## Risk

The probability of occurrence of an event. Calculated by dividing the number of events by the number of people at risk. See *Chapter 13*.

## Risk ratio, RR

The *risk* of an event happening in one group, divided by the risk of it happening in another group. See *Chapter 13*.

## ROC

Receiver Operator Characteristic (ROC): in a screening test, a cut-off value that gives an increase in sensitivity will give a decrease in specificity. A ROC curve is a graph showing the specificity and sensitivity for different possible values of the screening test. It helps us choose the test cut-off value that gives the best compromise between sensitivity and specificity.

## Sample

A small group drawn from a larger population.

## Sensitivity

This is the rate of pick-up of a condition in a test. In other words, the proportion of patients with the condition having a positive test result. See *Chapter 20*. Compare this with *specificity*.

## Significance

The probability of getting the results if the *null hypothesis* is true. See *Chapter 9*.

## Spearman rank correlation coefficient

An estimate of *correlation* used for *non-parametric variables*. See *Chapter 16*.

## Specificity

The rate of elimination of the possibility of disease by a test. In other words, the proportion of patients without the condition having a negative test result. See *Chapter 20*.

## Skewed data

A lack of symmetry in the *distribution* of data. See *Chapter 5*.

## Standard deviation, SD

A measure of the spread of scores away from the *mean*. See *Chapter 7*.

## Standard error of the mean

A measure of how close the *sample mean* is likely to be to the *population* mean.

## Statistical process control (SPC)

This is a statistical method for monitoring the quality of a process. It can give an early warning of when a measurement (e.g. a patient's blood glucose level) is changing and going outside a certain range.

## Stratified

A stratified *sample* is one that has been split into a number of subgroups.

## Student's *t* test

See *t test*.

## Subjects

The *sample* in a study.

## *t* test (also known as Student's *t* test)

The *t* test is a *parametric* test used to compare the *means* of two groups. See *Chapter 10*.

## Transformation

A transformation is where a mathematical formula is used to change the data. This will often be done to try to make the data follow a *normal distribution* so that a *parametric* test can be used. See *Chapter 10*.

## Two-tailed test

A test where the *null hypothesis* can be rejected whether the new treatment is better, or worse, than the current treatment. Compare this with a *one-tailed test*. See *Chapter 22.*

## Type I and II errors

Any statistical test can fail in two ways. A *hypothesis* that is correct can be rejected (type I error), or a hypothesis that is incorrect can be accepted (type II error). The chance of making a type I error is the same as the *P value.*

## Variable

Any characteristic that differs from subject to subject or time to time. In data analysis, variables may be called *fields* and refer to all the things recorded on the *cases.*

## Variance

A measure of the spread of scores away from the mean. It is the square of the *standard deviation.*

## Wilcoxon signed rank test

A *non-parametric* test for comparing the difference between paired groups, for instance before and after treatment. See *Chapter 11.*

## $\chi^2$ test

The chi-squared test is a test of association between two *categorical variables*. See *Chapter 12.*

## Yates' continuity correction

This is an adjustment to the *chi-squared* test to improve the accuracy of the *P value*. See *Chapter 12.*

# INDEX

(Page numbers in *italics* refer to the glossary)